Practising Yoga postures during pregnancy,
feeling of well-being through gentle and progressive
stretching and breathing exercises. A supple body, increased
muscle tone, deep breathing and relaxation can undoubtedly
increase a woman's chances of a successful pregnancy,
labour, delivery and a speedy return to fitness after the birth.

Sophy Hoare, eight months pregnant with her fourth
child, Max, during the photographing of postures for this
book, demonstrates the very real benefits of Yoga during
pregnancy and childbirth.

# Yoga and Pregnancy

SOPHY HOARE

UNWIN PAPERBACKS
London          Sydney

First published in Great Britain by Unwin Paperbacks 1985
Reprinted 1987

UNWIN HYMAN LIMITED
15–17 Broadwick Street
London W1V 1FP

Allen & Unwin Australia Pty Ltd
8 Napier Street, North Sydney, NSW 2060, Australia

Unwin Paperbacks with the Port Nicholson Press
60 Cambridge Terrace, Wellington, New Zealand

---

**British Library Cataloguing in Publication Data**

Hoare, Sophy
 Yoga and pregnancy.
 1. Prenatal care    2. Exercises for women
 3. Yoga, Hatha
 1. Title
 613.7′046    RG558.7
 ISBN 0–04–149061–4

---

Set in 11 on 13 point Times by
V & M Graphics Ltd, Aylesbury, Bucks
and printed in Great Britain by
Hazell Watson & Viney Limited,
Member of the BPCC Group,
Aylesbury, Bucks

*For Ros and Kathy, and Max*
*without whom this book would not have come about*

# Contents

# Acknowledgements

I would like to give love and thanks to all the teachers with whom I have studied, especially Penny Nield-Smith who introduced me to yoga; and to Sri B. K. S. Iyengar for all he has given us.

Love and thanks to my mother for giving me a positive attitude to birth, and to my husband and children for reinforcing it.

Special thanks to Kathy Hughes and Barbara Hicks for their help with the photographs in this book: Kathy supervising with a new baby in her arms, and Barbara modelling at seven months pregnant, on one of the hottest days of a hot summer.

Thanks also to the following women whose accounts of their own experiences appear in this book: Penny Cloutte, Stephanie Lambert, Tessa Turner, Tonie Greig, Kathy Hughes, Ros Claxton, Justyne Arnold, Amanda Webb, Sally Tagholm, Fran Crichton.

The yoga postures described in this book are based on the teaching of B. K. S. Iyengar.

Thanks are also due to Paul Ostrer who took the photographs, Laura McKechnie for the line drawings and Grafton Studios, London SW4 for the use of their exercise studio.

# Introduction

This is a time of changing attitudes towards birth; while in some areas the dependence on technology and professional medical skills seems to be reaching its height, in others a reaction to this trend is taking place and people are questioning many of the assumptions that have grown up around childbirth in our culture.

The seeds of this book were sown eleven years ago when I was in hospital after having our first child. I had been practising yoga for some years, as well as other forms of exercise such as judo, dance, swimming and running. I was very fit when I became pregnant and had a joyful and healthy pregnancy, continuing with yoga and swimming right up to the last day. I wanted a minimum of interference in the birth, having confidence in my body's ability to give birth naturally. I felt sure that it was in a fine condition for meeting the demands of birth, even though, like all mothers, I was apprehensive about the nature of the experience. It was after the birth that I noticed how valuable this confidence in my body had been. I had no stitches, my weight was back to normal two days after the birth, I had plenty of energy, plenty of milk and no problems breast-feeding. Any small post-natal problems I did have were due to my confinement in hospital for a week after the birth, and would not have occurred had I been at home.

All of this I took for granted, until I began to realise how different my experience was from that of the other women in my ward. There was not one who was free of problems. Most of them had had an episiotomy (a cut in the perineum) and were finding it difficult and painful to sit up and to clamber on and off their beds because of stitches. This made breast-feeding and caring for their babies in general a very trying experience. One had had a caesarian delivery and was in a lot of pain immediately after the operation and took days to take an interest in anything around her. Some had problems with constipation and the discomfort of suppositories and enemas. Others had problems with breast-feeding and were either taking drugs to suppress their milk because they had decided to bottle feed after all, or were using a breast pump on the nurses' advice to relieve engorgement, which only seemed to make matters worse. All women were shuffling dismally around the corridors, bent over, round shouldered, over-weight and flabby; some even still looked pregnant. All were in some way or other suffering.

What I gradually began to realise was that this was what was expected of them and by them: that pregnancy and birth were a kind of ordeal that it is women's lot to endure for the sake of their child, and that all the suffering that I was witnessing was regarded as *normal*. The women saw themselves as victims of their experience and dependent on medical care in matters concerning their own bodies and their relationship with their own children. This pointed to a lack of confidence in their own bodies and instincts, an alienation from their physical selves at a time when more than ever they needed to be in touch with their instincts for a safe and joyful experience and transition to motherhood.

As the years went by and I had more children and furthered my yoga practice, I clarified my own attitude more, becoming aware of the ways in which I had shared some of the assumptions inherent in our system. I began to see the far-reaching implications of our attitudes towards birth and our own confidence, or lack of it, in our bodies. To abandon responsibility for our own health and well-being, to leave the decisions to others, to the experts, is to lose our own sense of personal power, and, with it, our sense of connectedness to the rest of life and any real sense of joy and spiritual satisfaction. It means to live in a society where fear and mistrust are more prevalent than love and trust, where apathy and violence flourish. Pregnancy has become a disease, birth a hazardous obstetric operation and parenthood a burden; the negative aspects of these experiences have become central to our viewpoint. In his book, *Genèse de l'Homme Ecologique*, the French obstetrician Michel Odent writes:

> Whenever I am called on to talk about the conditions of birth, my reflections always stay within the framework of themes which are inherent in the system – themes such as the fight against pain, against risk, against violence and fear. I have never been asked to speak in terms of pleasure, hope, the revolutionary nature of love, or the origins of communication in man.

The way we approach and handle birth is not just a matter of a brief episode in our own and our children's lives, but is indicative of our whole attitude to life. A child's birth is the beginning of his or her relationship with others, with society, with the world, and the spirit in which it takes place sets the tone for the first years of life. The American writer Joseph Pearce has written with insight about the growth of the individual; he describes how, for development to continue, each phase must be relinquished for further growth, but that this is only possible where there has been a secure bonding with the previous phase or 'matrix':

> Once a knowledge of the matrix becomes a firm structure of knowing, that matrix must be separated from in some way, figuratively or literally, for a greater matrix, greater possibilities, and greater relations. That is, life must continually be given up for greater life, for as long as growth takes place.

He describes how this creative process is often disrupted by failure to bond to the universal matrices and how the individual's sense of personal power, of interaction with the life force, is supplanted by a bonding with and dependence on the particular culture.

> Cultural training ... enforces a bonding to culture. That is, the body of knowledge, with its institutions and priesthoods, becomes the surrogate matrix, presented to the child as the only safe space and source of strength and possibility, which, of course, the living earth alone actually is.

This conformity to culture, which can destroy confidence in one's own potential, begins for the individual with the parents' attitude to birth.

The function of yoga has traditionally been to cut through cultural dependence and bring the individual in touch with his or her own powers, to have faith in the truth that is found within. In this sense yoga is a revolutionary practice; for this reason it is a valuable tool for those who wish to discover their own ability to give birth, and who deplore the fact that we find it easier to trust electronic gadgetry and computers than we do our own bodies.

Yoga is about self-help. It breeds confidence and discrimination. It provides an excellent preparation for birth, encouraging a positive and healthy attitude. Pregnancy is indeed a special state in which the mother should take care of herself, but in our society this 'being careful' nearly always has a negative implication: don't eat too much or too little, don't overdo things, don't tire yourself, don't stretch your arms up above your head, don't do anything strenuous or acrobatic, don't take any risks. ... However, we cannot escape from the consequences of our actions by not doing, and we are not necessarily playing safe by not doing. In the case of pregnancy, refraining from exercise and over-protecting the body can be positively harmful. For example, the inverted postures stimulate the glands which control hormone production, thus protecting against miscarriage in the first months of pregnancy, a time when women are often advised to do nothing. Many postures strengthen the uterus, improving one's chances of a rapid, uncomplicated birth. And, perhaps most important of all, *not* doing encourages a negative and fearful attitude which can disturb the whole process of pregnancy and birth and cause complications, such is the close relationship between body and mind. Thus, it can be claimed that it is safer to practise yoga during pregnancy than not to do so. Improving your strength and health through yoga is to safeguard the healthy development of your child.

Of course, there are cases when caution must be exercised and professional advice sought, for example if there is a serious medical problem. But I believe that the majority of pregnant women need to be encouraged to develop their own bodily awareness and to trust in their instincts, and for this reason there are very few 'don'ts' in this book. All too often women give up yoga when they discover that they are pregnant, through ignorance and lack of faith in what their own body is telling them, or because their teacher is reluctant to keep them in their class. This is both sad and usually unnecessary – there is really no need for pregnant women to attend special yoga classes since for most of the time they can and should carry on with their normal practice. It is hoped that this book will help to reassure and inspire pregnant women and yoga teachers. I would like to conclude this introduction with a brief quotation from a French book on yoga and pregnancy by Ma Anand Gandha. Writing about squatting to give birth, as well as performing other natural functions, and talking generally of reviving our primitive, physical awareness, she says:

Il ne s'agit pas ici d'obscurantisme, ni de retour à la 'barbarie', mais il s'agit très simplement de sauver sa peau, et celle de son enfant. Si vous ne voulez pas qu'il naisse avec des lunettes et des béquilles, il s'agit de lui préparer un peu le terrain, et pour l'instant ce terrain c'est vous et vous seule.

(This is not a question of obscurantism, nor a return to barbarism, but a simple matter of survival – your own and that of your child. If you don't want your child to be born with spectacles and crutches, you have to prepare the ground a little, and for the time being that ground is you and you alone.)

## Chapter 1

# Yoga and Pregnancy: The Benefits

'I can describe yoga as being a very positive force in my own pregnancy. It was of enormous benefit and helped me to have a happy, contented nine months.'

*Kathy*

'The women's movement gave me a new way of understanding why and how I had so many negative feelings about my body and my sexuality, and new ways of resolving them. My pregnancy confirmed this process of reconciliation within me, a new confidence not just in my body, but also in the "Goddess within" – I feel I have made contact with a deeper layer of knowledge and wisdom about all sorts of things, not just about being a woman or how to cope with the various crises of motherhood and life. Doing yoga was a very important part of this process.

'One incident stands out in my memory. It was shortly after I had moved house. This was quite a difficult time for me, as I moved house several times in my childhood and I had only just become aware of how strong were the feelings which I was still carrying around about these long-past events ... I had suffered constantly from constipation during the year after my most traumatic move, and had only just come to see that this was the only way I had then of "holding on" to what I had lost. So I was in one way not surprised when a few weeks after moving this time, I was awoken by an agonising constipation pain. It was so acute that I could think only of how to relieve it. So I did an asana which I had in the past found helpful for constipation, and did some deep breathing, imagining my breath going to the centre of the pain and dissolving it. And it worked! Not all at once, and not simply by one asana, I had to try one or two other poses too – but I was by this means able to cure the pain. And while I was doing this the image of an ideal good mother came into my mind, as if she was telling me which positions to try, and when it was time to stop, to get back into bed and go to sleep. ... This incident gave me an enormously increased confidence in my ability to cope with the pain of labour, that I had the inner resources, both psychologically and practically, to cope with the pain.

'I don't mean that I thought that the pain of labour would be anything like that pain! But I was reassured in two ways. Firstly that pain could be modified on a physical level, by moving around and trying different positions and different breathing; and secondly, that I did have the inner resources to contact which would give me guidance as to how to find those different positions, about what I would need at the different stages.'

*Penny*

Central to this book is the idea of women taking responsibility for their own health. The day you start practising yoga, this is, in effect, what you are doing. Yoga is a path of self-development, a way of exploring your body and yourself in all its aspects, discovering your limitations and transcending them; it is a path of continuing and inevitable progress, whatever your age or state of health. Also, it leads to an awareness of, and a sense of oneness with, something greater than yourself, a source of energy and support which can be reached when we are able to let go of the fears, ambitions and desires which belong to the ego-self. Yoga is about building strength and firmness and about letting go; it is about taking responsibility for your own life and at the same time surrendering that responsibility when appropriate and simply trusting to life. Yoga cultivates strength and softness, stability and flexibility, responsibility and trust, a sense of independence and interdependence. For this reason yoga is ideally suited to pregnancy and birth, when the qualities of strength and endurance are needed as well as the ability to flow with a process that has taken over your body.

Childbirth is an intensely physical experience and even the least athletic, most cerebral woman cannot escape this fact. It is probably the most primitive and powerful physical experience any of us go through between our own birth and death. In our modern society most people's lives are physically undemanding. For many women pregnancy is the first time since childhood that they have become really aware of their body, and while some respond with joy and pleasure, others can be overwhelmed by it and feel burdened and afraid. For those in the latter category, it is all too easy to become 'medicalised', to become dependent on the doctor's professional care and to lose confidence in their own bodies and their ability to give birth naturally without medical intervention. Because of our cultural influences and the association of pregnancy with illness (ante-natal care and birth usually taking place in hospital), there are many women who go into labour doubting their own ability to give birth; and unless they receive loving care and support during labour, their own fear and lack of confidence can disturb the natural process to the extent that medical help becomes necessary. Marsden Wagner of the World Health Organization recounted the following anecdote in his talk at the London Active Birth conference:

'I attended a homebirth in Copenhagen of a woman having her first child. . . .

2

It was clear that the woman and her husband ... immediately began shoving the primary responsibility for the whole affair on to the midwife. Susanne, in a very slow and subtle way, assisted the woman during the first stage from a dependent role to an independent role. Indeed, the first stage, in my mind, could be best described by the woman asking herself again and again 'Can I do it?'. ... As the bearing down rushes came and she could herself feel the descending child, (she had had absolutely no anaesthesia of any kind) she suddenly got a look on her face right in the middle of a rush and called out in a triumphant voice, "Jeg kan klare det." (I can do it.) A look of ecstasy swept over her face and her rapidly increased self-control and self-realisation and self-fulfilment was palpable. This woman had the opportunity to experience the power and control of her own body. ... When Susanne asked me for my impression afterwards, I said to her, "It is so beautiful, it is so powerful, and, my God, it is so simple."'

The woman who is healthy and fit, who feels responsible for her own health and at one with her body, is most likely to have a positive and joyful experience of pregnancy and birth and to adapt without difficulty to life as a new mother.

The beauty of yoga is that it is a discipline not only of the body but of the whole person; it encompasses physical, emotional, mental and spiritual health. According to yoga, the body is the temple of the soul and should be neither neglected nor pampered. Whatever our personal leanings, yoga always helps to redress the balance in ourselves. For those who are not drawn to sport or other physical exercise, yoga is an ideal way of learning to live freely and fully in the body since its approach is at the same time gentle and direct. If you try any of the simplest yoga stretches you feel immediately different about yourself; it is as if you have shifted nearer to your centre, as if you and your body have become one. The benefits of yoga can be experienced immediately, even by the beginner who has done little or no exercise before. For those who practise a sport or other form of exercise, yoga provides a complementary activity since it stretches and loosens muscles which become tight through repetitive use (a typical example being the hamstring muscles which shorten with regular running, cycling, or even walking). Yoga stretching helps to undo resistance and 'open' the body and the mind, a very valuable preparation for childbirth.

There is a special need for exercise during pregnancy since extra demands are made on the body from the very beginning. During the early stages, the volume of blood pumped by the heart is increased considerably to supply the womb with the materials necessary for building the new life. Ligaments and joints soften and loosen to make more space in the body, and need the protection of well-toned muscles. Towards the end, the body has to carry up to two stones extra weight, putting more strain than usual on the lower back if posture and muscle tone are poor. During labour itself the body has to withstand the intense and sometimes prolonged activity of the uterus, the largest muscle in the human body. And during the post-natal period the changes which take place in the mother's body and life-style are very sudden, requiring resilience to ride them smoothly.

The yoga postures in this book will bring innumerable benefits to the pregnant woman. They build strength in the legs and back and help to develop strong, healthy feet. At the same time they create an awareness of good posture, bringing the whole body into alignment. This combination of strength and balance is extremely important during pregnancy, when the extra weight carried in front often distorts posture, causing fatigue and pain from permanent tension. The weakness which arises from bad posture and lack of exercise can lead to problems (especially in the back) which can persist for long after the baby is born. All the postures stretch and strengthen the spine thoroughly and evenly. Improving circulation to the spine affects the entire body, since the nerves have their origin in the spinal column.

Muscle strength is also important during pregnancy to protect the joints, whose ligaments become looser than usual under the influence of increased hormone production. The great advantage of yoga in this respect is that it strengthens without tightening; it increases the suppleness that is necessary for birth while protecting against over-stretching (as long as it is practised with sensitivity and without forcing). As the joints become more mobile, positions that are useful during pregnancy and birth (for example, squatting and sitting cross-legged) can be assumed with ease. The yoga postures also open the chest, freeing the lungs and heart from unnecessary pressure due to bad posture, and facilitating good deep breathing, vital for the baby's healthy growth. Circulation is therefore improved together with any associated problems. As well as the more visible benefits, yoga improves and regulates the functioning of the internal organs, glands and nerves. In fact, most of the ailments that our society considers normal during pregnancy are quite unnecessary!

The woman who has explored her body through yoga practice is likely to feel free during pregnancy and labour to follow the dictates of her body rather than those of convention, finding the appropriate posture for each situation. In this way she grows steadily more in touch with her body and her instincts and handles herself with a grace and ease which are far removed from the awkward, cumbersome figures that many pregnant women become in the later stages of pregnancy. Carrying the baby is experienced not as a burden, but as an enormous privilege and the joy that this brings is bound to affect the mother's relationship with her baby.

Confidence in the way your body works is an outstanding advantage in labour, when you have to let the body take over completely, to trust that it 'knows what it is doing' in the face of powerful and often painful and overwhelming sensations. This is especially true of a first birth, when a mother is more likely to be apprehensive and tense, but it may also happen that the experience of a subsequent birth is so different from the first that you are equally unprepared for it. The process of yoga stretching provides a good preparation for accepting the experience of birth. Although the sensations of childbirth are far more intense than those encountered in yoga practice, the ability to relax into the stretching sensation that is learnt in yoga is entirely relevant to birth. Yoga teaches you to discriminate between the 'positive' pain of stretching and the 'negative' pain of injury. When practising the yoga postures you come up against pain continually, learning how to listen to the pain, to meet it instead of tensing against it, in order to respond in a way which dissolves it. Injury in yoga happens only when you stop listening to your body, so it is really possible to learn through yoga how to tune into the body.

All this requires a great deal of concentration, to make the mind very still and receptive. Hatha yoga is a form of meditation in action. This meditative state of mind is just what is needed for the body to function smoothly during birth. It is this altered state of consciousness that Dr Michel Odent talks about and tries to encourage in his maternity unit in Pithiviers, France, by adjusting the environment in which women give birth. He provides a birth room (which he calls the 'primitive room') in which the colours are muted, there is semi-darkness, there is the opportunity to play music, there is no furniture except a platform with cushions, so that women feel free to take up any position they like. A commonly used posture for the most difficult stage of labour is the kneeling position, which Michel Odent points out is the position of prayer, a form of meditation. In addition, the attendants at the birth communicate with the mother chiefly by touch, deliberately avoiding conversation, which tends to disturb the meditative state of mind by making demands on the active, rational brain. And, for those mothers who want it, or who have difficulty in relaxing, there are pools of warm water in which they can immerse themselves completely. It has been found that immersion in warm water produces the same brain pattern as meditation.

Now, most women today are going into labour in conditions very different from those at Pithiviers. Hospitals are bright, harsh, noisy places; labour wards can be full of people coming and going, delivery beds do not invite freedom of movement, and you may have to deal with doctors who are complete strangers continually bombarding you with questions or instructions. So it is clearly a great advantage for a woman, when conditions are not ideal, to be used to turning her attention inwards, through yoga practice, and to find a place within herself where she is distracted as little as possible by obtrusive external stimuli. Moreover, she needs to be in a state of mind in which she is unconcerned about what other people think of her or what sort of behaviour is expected of her. She must be able to do whatever her instincts tell her, whether this means shouting or moaning, or rocking her body to and fro. In other words, essential to the altered, primitive state of consciousness is a kind of social de-conditioning. This probably comes more easily to those who practise yoga, because they have become accustomed to relying on their own intuition and judgement rather than on what other people tell them. Yoga helps to undo, or at least loosen, a certain amount of our cultural conditioning, which, in our society, tends to take us away from the physical and the primitive.

When citing the benefits of practising yoga during pregnancy, there is a danger of presenting yoga as a kind of magic formula which will ensure a problem-free pregnancy and an easy birth, but this is not so. Yoga is not a means to an end, but a continuing life process of exploration which transforms our attitudes to ourselves and the world. It is a way of working with ourselves in order to live life skilfully and harmoniously, and to retain equanimity, a sense of our unchanging centre, in the face of any circumstances. In the words of the teacher B. K. S. Iyengar, 'If the foundation is firm, the building can withstand calamities. The practice of yoga is the foundation, so that the self is not shaken under any circumstances.'

Of course, working on yourself will influence what happens to you. Being fit and healthy optimises your chances of a happy pregnancy and birth; a relaxed and positive attitude communicates itself to other people, so influencing their actions, however subtly. The repercussions of our own behaviour are far reaching, if largely unknowable. So, by practising yoga you are assuming responsibility for yourself and reducing your dependence on others and your vulnerability to external conditions. When problems do arise, you may find within yourself the resources to deal with them. For example, you may experience some physical problem during pregnancy or the breast-feeding period and find that instinctively you know what action to take, whether it is exercise or rest, increasing your fluid intake or changing your diet – it is surprising how often our bodies will reveal the right course of action if we only listen to them, and heal themselves if we place our trust in them. Paradoxically, the more we take responsibility for ourselves and become independent, the more we experience the interdependence of all things and are able to trust in the natural process and in other people, including our professional care-givers. And a relationship of trust with these people is essential for an undisturbed, natural birth.

So, yoga is a way of 'preparing the ground' from within. It is an ideal preparation for a natural birth and a way of equipping yourself to deal with the unexpected, for every birth experience is different and, for all the careful planning, cannot be predicted; you have to be ready to venture into the unknown.

*Chapter 2*

# How Much Should You Do?

'I had an unusually eventful and stressful childbearing year. But fortunately I was very well throughout. Apart from a little nausea when I was hungry in the early weeks, I felt very well and was active up to the end. Even during my labour, which started very slowly, I went for walks, belly-danced, made chutney and beat my partner at cards! I rode my bike up to the middle of my eighth month, and gave up then for lack of the aggression and concentration needed to survive London's traffic on a bicycle rather than for lack of physical energy.'

*Penny*

'I was already pregnant when I joined a yoga class and was immediately pleased by the changes I felt. Firstly, it was not a physical response so much as an emotional one that impressed me. As a pregnant woman one gets used to being treated as a sick person – a victim – many decisions seem to be made in spite of one's desires and gradually it becomes easy to succumb to the wishes of specialists, doctors, etc. By beginning a yoga class I had started to take on responsibility for my own healthy pregnancy and was astonished by what my "lumpy body" could achieve without strain. Even a well informed mother-to-be is subjected to myths and superstitions about pregnancy from all sides, so I had been hesitant to try some positions. With confidence in my teacher's knowledge, I was able to dispel many such fears and find that my body was much stronger and healthier than I had realised. This confidence developed to the point where I felt stronger to make decisions about the labour I wanted and press for freedoms of movement that I might not otherwise have felt I could reasonably expect.'

*Tonie*

Yoga can be practised all the way through pregnancy, labour and the post-natal period, because it can be adapted to suit each individual's needs and there is always a suitable posture for every situation. Yoga teaches us how to face up to every situation positively, so in this general sense it can be practised safely by anyone at any time. More specifically, women like to know which yoga postures are especially suitable for pregnancy and whether there are any that are dangerous. While it is possible to list a number of basic postures which have particular benefits

7

for the pregnant woman (and it is these which are included in this book), there are no hard and fast rules about what should not be done. The limitations imposed by pregnancy vary considerably from one person to another, depending on individual fitness and experience. In general, as long as you practise in the right spirit, it is wise to follow your own body. All the principles which should underlie your practice at other times apply even more during pregnancy. For example, the yoga postures are designed to create space in the body, and sometimes more space is made and a healthier stretch gained by modifying the standard pose, perhaps moving into a half-way position instead of completing it. It is even more important to work in this way during pregnancy, when making space is essential for the well-being of the baby as well as yourself. As long as your attitude is right you will not do any damage. Listen to your own body very carefully. Do not let the rapport with your body be disturbed by fear or anxiety that a particular exercise may not be safe; simply proceed carefully with a positive attitude and your body will tell you if and when you should stop. Equally, do not try to prove to yourself that you can still do everything regardless of the pregnancy – where there are limitations they must be accepted. If you let yourself be guided by the head rather than the body, this is the only way you are likely to do yourself any harm, through neglect or injury. Try thinking of yourself as a yoga student who happens to be pregnant rather than a pregnant woman doing yoga.

It is possible to start yoga at any time during pregnancy, although the later you start the fewer poses you will be able to attempt. Those who have been practising yoga for some time before becoming pregnant will obviously be able to do a greater variety of postures for longer than a beginner. However, although the earlier you start the better (ideally before conception), it is never too late, and you and the baby can only benefit from practising the asanas. After all, if you practised only Tadasana, the basic standing posture, you would improve your posture and become healthier and more relaxed as a result. If you are a beginner in yoga you can follow the guidelines laid down in this book. Most of the postures illustrated are simple, basic ones that can safely be attempted by anyone; a few should not be done by beginners, and this is made clear in the instructions. The asanas have been selected for having special benefits for pregnancy and between them they form an excellent regular programme. If you are a more advanced student, you can continue practising a wider range of postures if you wish – for example, some of the more advanced back bends can be continued into the eighth month if correctly done – but if you are as experienced as this you will be able to judge for yourself how much you can do. For the student of average experience, nearly all the postures in this book can be done to the end of pregnancy. Beginners should concentrate on the standing poses and the sitting poses, which will give strength, flexibility and postural awareness.

Make sure that your yoga programme during pregnancy includes regular practice of the standing postures, the basic sitting poses and inverted poses (though beginners should get help with the latter). The standing postures should be done at least twice a week to build up strength and endurance, to gain a sense of being grounded and stable, and to improve breathing and circulation. The basic sitting postures can easily be incorporated into your everyday life, in which case you need not make a special time to practise them, except when using them for deep breathing or meditation. You could cultivate the habit of sitting on the floor instead of chairs whenever possible. This is in any case the most comfortable way of sitting in the later months of pregnancy, since your spine can stretch up evenly from the pelvis, avoiding backache and making plenty of space in the front of the body so that the abdomen does not feel heavy or squashed; and breathing is unhampered. If you are sitting for long periods, place a cushion, wedge or folded blanket under the back of the buttocks and if you want support, sit against a wall. If you are writing or typing, it can be much more comfortable to settle yourself on the floor and work at a low table such as a coffee table. When helping or talking to young children, it is a good idea to come down to their level by squatting or kneeling on the ground beside them. In fact, whenever you find yourself bending uncomfortably from the waist to perform a task, think instead of dropping on to one knee, kneeling on both knees or perhaps squatting; this is much better for the back and helps to keep your joints flexible.

Squatting is an excellent way of resting if you have to stand for long periods, for example, waiting for buses or queueing. It instantly relieves aches in the small of the back and avoids the heavy, downward dragging feeling that often comes with standing still during pregnancy. If you cannot go into a full squat it is well worth practising at home with support until you can rest your heels comfortably on the ground. When doing housework, such as sweeping or washing floors, get on to your hands and knees whenever possible rather than standing and bending at the waist. The all-fours position is extremely comfortable during pregnancy, since it takes the weight of the uterus off the spine, pelvis and legs; it is also a very stable working position in which you can work vigorously without strain. There are many examples of situations in everyday life in which you can use your body well with just a little awareness, even if it does not strictly conform to the social norm. The more yoga you do, the more your bodily awareness increases and the more you will eschew those aspects of our civilisation which tend to dull this awareness (the most simple example being 'comfortable' soft chairs).

Do not over-protect your body. You can be just as active during pregnancy as at any other time, although your *pace* of life will almost certainly slow down. It is your rhythm which changes rather than your energy level (with the exception of the fatigue often felt in the first two or three months), and it is important to listen to your own inner rhythm for a healthy, stress-free pregnancy. This is another reason why yoga is so suitable at this time. In yoga you cannot be in a hurry. Rushing through the postures with an eye on the clock is not yoga. While practising the asanas you have to keep your attention fully on what is going on in your body and your mind, observing your own reactions; in other words, you are totally in the present moment, with no mental idea of achieving or moving towards a future goal. It is a process of growing and unfolding rather than forcing, and is thus a process which has close affinities with that of pregnancy, birth and childhood. The happiest and healthiest pregnancies are perhaps those in which every stage is enjoyed for itself, rather than those which are seen as a period which has to be endured for the sake of a future product – the child. Women who feel this way instinctively about their pregnancy will find yoga a natural and appropriate activity. Those who are less at ease with their pregnant state will find that yoga helps to give them this ease by bringing them in touch with their own body and hence with the growing baby.

## Hints on practice

The Sanskrit word for yoga posture, Asana, means literally seat. This implies that the postures are to be held with steadiness and ease. They need to be held long enough for the body to accept the position and begin to relax into it. If you reach the point where it is a strain to continue holding a position, then you should stop and rest briefly before continuing with the next one. You should never force the body in yoga, and this is especially important during pregnancy. Breathing should never be difficult or strained. Never hold your breath, either while moving into a pose or while maintaining it. Concentrate especially on the exhalation, releasing any tightness that you are aware of with the out breath. In this way you use the breath to help undo the tensions which are standing between you and complete freedom of movement. Your practice should always leave you feeling good – healthy, balanced and refreshed. If you feel drained or exhausted after certain asanas, this is a sign that they should be discontinued or approached in a different way. Always leave time for relaxation in Savasana, the Corpse Pose, at the end of your practice, or you will not experience the full benefits of yoga; instead of feeling calm and refreshed you could feel slightly irritable.

If possible, practise at the same time each day, even if the length of time you practise differs. Morning and early evening are good times. Do not practise on a full stomach – several hours should have elapsed since a full meal. Try to have a special place in the house for your yoga practice which is clean, warm, airy and pleasant to be in; in the summer you may like to use the garden. Clothes should be completely unrestricting, so wear as little as possible while being comfortably warm. You should always work with bare feet. The feet need to be able to make sensitive contact with the ground when standing and with the air when sitting or in the inverted postures. Also, the toes should be able to spread out wide, and even wearing socks inhibits the action of the feet to a great extent. Cotton footless tights in an extra large size and cotton tee-shirts are very comfortable.

You will see in the illustrations that various pieces of equipment are useful for encouraging a good stretch. The first of these is an area of wall-space, wide enough to stretch your arms out horizontally against it. This is useful for both the standing and sitting poses and it is important to be able to move right up against it, so do not choose a wall with radiators or other immovable objects in the way. Most of the other items should be easy to find around the house: a chair, a low stool, a strong, firm belt, a brick or a block of wood (or a couple of thick books), cushions, and a blanket or two. Rather more specialist pieces of equipment are a long pole (a piece of thick dowelling is ideal), a short heavy stick and a wedge for sitting on. These are not essential for your practice, but they can be very useful.

Remember to vary your routine a little so that it does not become mechanical, and listen to your body as to what type of postures and how much you do on any particular day. Do not go on working when your body is tired, but relax deeply in Savasana. As your pregnancy progresses, the nature of your practice will undoubtedly change, with the number of asanas that you practise regularly becoming fewer, but the quality of your practice can continue to become ever finer and more precise.

*Chapter 3*

# The Standing Postures

'Physically, the effects of yoga were surprisingly immediate. Conditions such as swollen feet, tired legs, piles, responded to specific yoga exercises, and the major change of being taught to stand correctly meant that many problems involving backache and strain were relieved considerably.

The preparations thus made did affect the labour itself on many levels. I felt strong and positive so that although the onset of labour was dramatic and intense, I was able to gain control very quickly and did not get overwhelmed. The standing postures had given me strength to move about and I was also able to adopt many more unconventional postures without embarrassment, so that I could constantly change position to cope with the labour. If you are used to a yoga class where you may end up in many potentially "undignified" positions, the "basicness" of labour is easier to handle as you learn to be unashamed of your body and able to "listen" to what it can cope with.'

*Tonie*

When you are pregnant, the standing postures form the mainstay of your yoga practice, whether you are an experienced student or a complete beginner. The standing postures give you a firm foundation for carrying the growing baby and your own extra weight with ease and pleasure. They help to activate and ground the feet, they strengthen the legs and ankles, bring mobility to the hips and spine as well as the shoulders and neck, and train the body in correct posture. Bad posture is the cause of many of the weaknesses which arise during pregnancy, especially back problems. The standing postures also help to increase energy and reduce fatigue, partly by working the body hard and developing stamina, partly by bringing the body into better alignment so that unnecessary tension is eliminated.

The importance of strong legs must be emphasised here. The general sense of tiredness that many women seem to experience may be largely due to weakness in the legs and feet, for it is noticeable how often beginners in yoga find it hard to stand firmly on their two feet for any length of time – knees and ankles begin to give way and muscles to shake. However, yoga does not give a hard, sinewy, unyielding strength of the type keen runners or cyclists might develop; it encourages the leg muscles to lengthen and soften and the joints to become more mobile. Lengthening the hamstring muscles in the back of the legs helps to release the lower back, an area of weakness in human beings generally, and even more vulnerable in pregnancy.

Finally, the standing poses stretch and open the whole body, creating more space for the baby and the internal organs; the ribs are able to expand freely, facilitating deep breathing and improving the mother and baby's circulation, and reducing pressure and strain on the lungs and heart. The breathlessness and heartburn that is often experienced in later pregnancy can be helped considerably by improving posture.

## The basic stretches

The positions illustrated on the following pages are ideal for the beginning of your practice. They progressively stretch the legs and spine, 'ground' the feet, flex the hip joints and generally make the whole body feel more open and alive. Beginners should do only the positions shown in the first two pictures.

### Hamstring stretch

This stretch, and the next one, can be done at any time around the house when you have a few seconds to spare. All you need is a table, steady chair, windowsill or chest of drawers to rest the raised heel on. You need to find a support that is just the right height for you, depending on how stiff you are. Do not start too high; your support should be high enough to give you a definite feeling of stretch in the back of the legs, but not so high that you cannot maintain a stable, upright posture with both knees quite straight. Your normal standing position (as in Tadasana, p. 19) should be barely disturbed by raising one leg. The standing foot should take your weight evenly and firmly, and from the firm contact of that foot with the ground your whole body should be able to stretch up freely (Fig. 3.1).

The position of the hips should not be disturbed when you raise one leg; the rear view shows how the buttocks should stay level with each other (there is usually a tendency for the buttock of the raised leg to lift, throwing the body out of balance). The side view shows how the supporting leg should be perpendicular to the floor, hip above heel, so make sure that you are the correct distance from your support. The raised leg should rest on the centre back of the heel, so that your toes and kneecap face upwards. If you feel wobbly or unbalanced, find something lower to rest your heel on. With practice, you will be able to raise your leg higher, though there will come a time in later pregnancy when you will be limited by the size of your abdomen.

The variation with the arms stretched above the head is especially good during pregnancy, since it really opens the front of the body and makes space for the baby to move and stretch. However, if you feel dizzy when you raise your arms, place your hands on your hips instead; this also helps you to feel whether your hips are properly aligned.

13

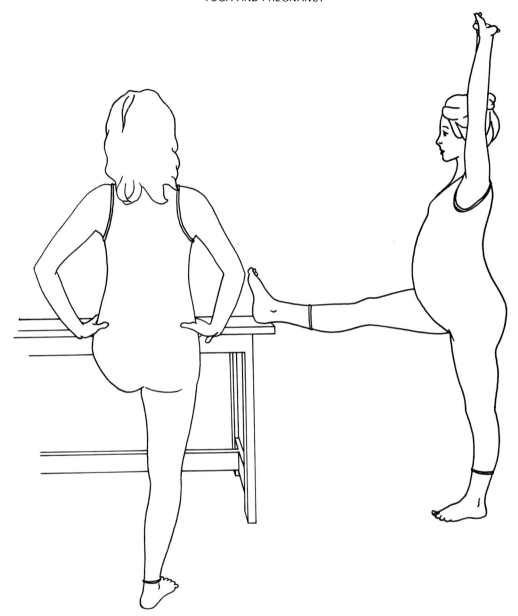

**3.1**  Hamstring stretch

Alternate the position of the legs, and hold for an equal length of time on each side.

## Spine stretch 1

Find something to rest on which is about hip height. Here (see Fig. 3.2 back figure),

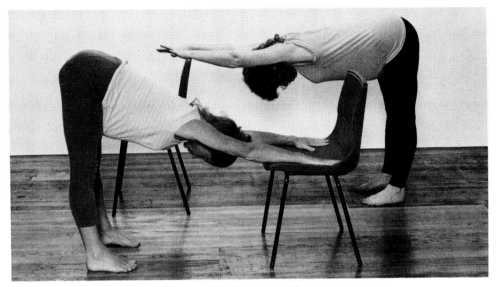

**3.2** Spine stretches

the back of a chair is used, but a work-top, shelf or just the wall would do equally well. Stand with your feet parallel to each other, hip width apart. Make sure that you are the right distance away from the support – just far enough to be able to reach out and rest your hands on it with straight arms and back, keeping your legs perpendicular. Plant your feet firmly on the ground, spreading the toes and lifting the inner arches, and keep your legs straight, lengthening the backs of the legs from heels to hips by lifting the buttock bones. Rest your hands lightly, with arms outstretched, looking at the ground so that the back of your neck is parallel to it, in line with the rest of your spine. Do not tense your wrists, arms or shoulders; try to release the shoulder and upper back area, widening the space between your neck and shoulders and letting your lower neck and upper back release downwards towards the ground, opening the chest. Use the exhalation to help you let go here.

Now concentrate on flattening and lengthening the rest of your back. As you inhale, feel your back broadening out from your spine, and on the exhalation let your spine lengthen, stretching out of the pelvis, by drawing your buttock bones away from your head. Your whole back should be flat, parallel to the ground; if in doubt, feel your spine with one hand to find out whether there are any humps. Equally, there should be no hollow in the small of the back, so make sure that you are not concave in that area. This is especially important during pregnancy, when the lumbar curve is more pronounced than usual. Concentrate only on lengthening the spine, trying to spread the buttock bones apart as you draw them back. As your spine stretches, you may need to move your feet back slightly to keep them in line with your hips, legs perpendicular.

This simple but extremely effective stretch can be done at any time when you feel in need of revitalisation. A good opportunity is when working in the kitchen, since sinks and work tops are a good height for placing the hands on.

15

## Spine stretch 2

A chair is ideal for this stretch, which is a continuation of the previous one and a good preparation for the Dog Pose (Svanasana), shown in the next picture. This position is also a good substitute for Svanasana for beginners, or those who find Svanasana difficult at the end of pregnancy.

For stability, push your chair against the wall. Working in exactly the same way as in the last exercise, reach out with your hands on to the back of the chair seat (as shown in Fig. 3.2, front). As before, check that your feet are parallel, hip width apart, and that your legs are straight, with your hips directly above your feet. Lift your buttock bones high, so that you are able to keep your whole spine, from pelvis to back of neck, in one smooth, straight line, letting it 'grow' out of the hips. Make sure that you are not tensing your shoulders, neck or hands. The front of your body should be perfectly free and open and you should be able to breathe deeply and easily, releasing the spine on every exhalation. In later pregnancy you will appreciate these spine stretches for the way in which they take the weight of the baby off the spine and pelvis.

## Padangusthasana (Big Toe Catch) and Adho Mukha Svanasana (Downward Facing Dog Pose)

These two yoga postures continue the forward-bending action started in the previous spine stretches. They can both be practised right to the end of pregnancy, but only by those who can bend easily from the hips, keeping their spine long and straight. If your back is not flat when you do spine stretch 2 with your hands on the chair, then do not try to take your hands to the floor.

To practise *Padangusthasana* (Fig. 3.3, left), stand with your feet parallel, hip

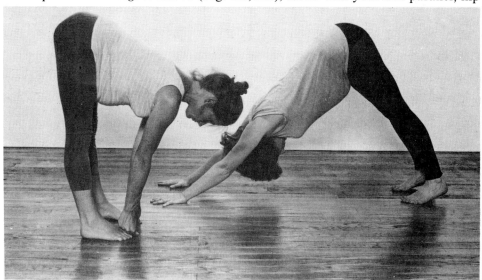

**3.3**  Padangusthasana (left) and Adho Mukha Svanasana (right)

16

width apart. Plant your feet firmly on the ground, keeping them 'alive', and bend forward carefully from the hips, lifting your buttock bones and releasing the muscles in the back of the legs. As you bend forward, place your hands on your belly and lift it forward with you, making as much space as possible between the groin and the navel. This prevents the abdomen and uterus from being squashed against the thighs. You will feel at what stage of your pregnancy it is necessary to use the hands in this way. With the first two fingers (thumbs turned outwards), pick up your big toes. Continue to lift and spread the buttock bones and let the spine lengthen. Keep your awareness very much in your feet, legs and hips, and do not let the upper part of your body become hard or tight. Be firm in the legs and soft in the upper body. Press your big toe joints firmly into the floor. Keep the back of your neck in line with the spine.

Breathe normally and hold the pose for as long as is comfortable. Then come up to the standing position while inhaling, lifting your head first and unbending from the hips; the hips are the hinge, enabling your back to stay straight throughout.

To practise *Svanasana* (Fig. 3.3, right), start on all fours. Have your knees and feet hip width apart and your toes tucked under. Place your hands carefully and squarely on the ground just under your shoulders. The middle fingers should be pointing directly forwards, the other fingers and the thumbs spreading as far as possible away from them. Make sure that your index fingers are pressing down firmly – there is often a tendency for the inner edge of the hand to lift up from the floor. With an exhalation, straighten your legs so that you are standing on your toes, lifting your hips up and back away from your head. Your arms should stay straight all the time. Lift your buttock bones as high as you possibly can, making a long straight line from wrists to hips, and keeping your heels up to increase the lift of the hips. At this point, if your belly feels squashed, you can use one hand to lift it forward out of the way of the thighs. Now, with both hands firmly on the floor, and without losing the height you have gained in the hips and groins, gradually press your heels down to the ground. If you can touch the ground with your heels, stand firmly on your feet, taking the weight on the heels, lifting the arches and spreading the toes. Keep the arches lifted, even if your heels do not rest flat on the floor. If your heels are a long way from the ground, place a block or thick book under them so that you have something to press on. If your calf muscles are tight, practise the squatting position frequently to help stretch them.

The outer shoulders and outer hips should be firm and the spine should be quiet and flat, lengthening on every exhalation. Stiff areas of the back will show up as bumpy vertebrae; very supple people should beware of collapsing and hollowing the lumbar spine. If you have someone to help you, get them to place a length of stick along your spine (like the one shown on p. 20), and try to touch the stick all the way along, from neck to tail-bone.

If this pose feels restful, it can be held for quite a long time. But if you find it tiring, hold it for short periods and relax in the all fours position in between. A good way to relax after practising Svanasana is in the 'Frog' Pose, shown on p. 53.

# The feet

Before continuing with the rest of the postures, it is necessary to consider the feet. The feet are the foundation of good posture, and having strong, supple feet will help you to carry your baby with ease and grace throughout your pregnancy. Try to walk barefoot as often as possible, walking on rough ground as well as smooth. Let your feet become sensitive to different textures. It can be just as pleasurable to tread on knobbly concrete or coconut matting as on soft sand or carpet. Learn to pick up small objects with your toes (this will prove extremely useful later on when you have a baby in your arms and you need to retrieve something from the floor!). Sometimes, when you are sitting down, use your hands to bend and stretch the toes passively in all directions. Try taking each toe in turn and flexing it as far as possible towards the sole of the foot, then extending it in the opposite direction, then pulling it out away from the foot, running thumb and finger from the base to the tip of the toe (rather like pulling a ring off a finger). Then use your hands to spread your toes apart from each other, keeping the toes quite relaxed.

You can also try rolling the foot over a thick baton or milk bottle. To exercise the ankles, practise rotating your feet from the ankle joint, first clockwise then anti-clockwise, flexing and extending fully as you circle them. Squatting and kneeling (in Virasana, Hero Pose) are both excellent postures for strengthening and suppling the feet and ankles.

When you have to wear shoes, make sure that there is plenty of room for your toes to spread out comfortably (this also applies to socks and tights). Wear high heels rarely if at all, since they shorten the Achilles tendon and calf muscle and distort your posture by throwing your weight too far forward. This is particularly undesirable during pregnancy when there is additional weight at the front of the body already pulling you forward and a tendency to hollow back and slack stomach muscles. Make it a habit to become aware of your feet from time to time during the day – this is easier if you discard your shoes. Really experience the ground under your feet and imagine that you are drawing up energy from the earth to stabilise and centre you. You will notice that it then becomes easier to release any tension you may have in your upper body, especially shoulders, upper back, neck and hands. The feet affect the whole body. This habit will be very useful after your baby is born, when you may find yourself becoming tense in your shoulders and arms from carrying the baby and from pushing prams and push-chairs.

When practising the standing postures, always work with bare feet. Learn to stand properly in Tadasana (Mountain Pose) with your weight evenly balanced on both feet before attempting those postures in which you balance on one leg. Keep the soles of your feet sensitive to the ground beneath them. Spread out your toes as much as you can, making sure that they are not tense or curled under; your toes should be relaxed but firmly planted. Always keep the arches of the feet lifted; spreading the toes and pressing the base of the toes to the ground helps to do this – do not let the inner arches collapse so that the feet roll inwards.

Some beginners in yoga have lifeless feet with collapsed arches, and toes that seem to be sandwiched together in one lump; others have tense feet with toes curled rigidly as if trying to cling on to or evade the floor. Either way, your body cannot be well supported and aligned and there will be no sense of stability or confidence. When you stand on the ground, try imagining that your feet have roots going deep into the earth. Imagine also a two-way give and take between you and the ground: the feet feel the ground and the ground feels your feet upon it; the feet press downwards with your weight and at the same time draw energy upwards from the earth. When you become aware of your feet in this way, you may notice your whole posture subtly changing.

## Basic standing postures

### Tadasana, Mountain Pose

Tadasana is the basic standing posture, to which one returns after each of the other standing poses, and it forms the basis of our posture for everyday life. Tadasana should be practised as often as possible during pregnancy, when the weight of the baby encourages a common form of bad posture: the hollow-backed, round-shouldered slump. The lower back tends to curve excessively to compensate for the extra weight in front, particularly when the abdominal and buttock muscles are not firm. The protruding abdomen pulls forward more and more, further weakening the sagging stomach muscles and putting great strain on the spine. The key to adjusting this fault is the position of the pelvis, which should remain centred and level rather than tipping forward. To adjust the pelvis, take the tail-bone towards the floor and lift the front hip bones slightly. If you place your thumbs and forefingers of each hand on the back and front of the upper pelvis, you will be able to feel the bones which form the top of the pelvic basin at front and back and to judge whether they are level or not. Get used to tilting the pelvis gently to and fro, experimenting with it until you are familiar with the feeling of it in the neutral position compared with the tipped positions. As you alter the position of the pelvis, notice the effect this has on the legs and spine.

To practise Tadasana, stand with your feet hip width apart (see Fig. 3.4). Your feet should be parallel and firmly planted on the ground, as described above. Make sure that your weight is balanced evenly between your two feet and between the heel and the ball of each foot. Spread your toes out, lift the inner arches of the feet and lift also the inner and outer ankles and the shin bones. From the firm downward pressure of the feet on the ground, there should be a feeling of lifting up actively through the rest of the body. Stretch your legs up, keeping your kneecaps lifted so that they flatten into the legs, and at the same time lift the front hip bones very slightly so that the tail-bone moves downwards. You should get a feeling in the legs and pelvis of being stable and firmly grounded; from this stability in the lower body, the spine can stretch up freely. Notice how the lower spine lengthens when you adjust the pelvis and move the tail-bone down. Feel the whole spine

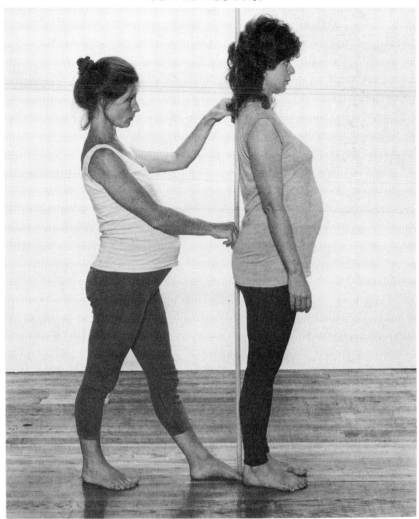

**3.4** Tadasana, with pole

lengthening and growing upwards to the crown of the head, and feel the rib-cage lifting away from the pelvis. You are making more space in the trunk for the baby to grow and move, for the lungs to breathe deeply, and for the heart and other internal organs to function more easily. Stretching removes pressure and tension.

As you lift the ribs and spine, make sure that you do not lift the shoulders too. Your shoulders should drop down and back away from your ears, as if being pulled down by the weight of the forearms. Let your arms and hands hang loosely from your shoulders and make sure that your wrists and hands are relaxed. Your breast-bone should be lifting straight up without protruding aggressively forwards. Keep your feeling of centre in the pelvis and let the trunk grow up from there without distortion. Your shoulders relax down as your neck stretches up, creating more space between your shoulders and your ears. Let your head balance lightly above your shoulders.

Ankles, hips, shoulders and ears should all be in one vertical line. The illustration shows Tadasana from the side (see Fig. 3.4), and also shows a way of checking your alignment. Here, a length of thick dowelling is used. Your helper places the bottom of the pole between your heels. You can then adjust the pelvis so as to reduce any excessive curve in the lumbar spine. The sacrum (back of pelvis) and the back of the head should touch the pole. Let your whole spine 'grow' up the pole to the crown of your head. If you have no one to help you, you can do this on your own by standing against an outer corner where two walls meet.

Learning to stand in Tadasana can make you an inch or so taller if your posture was bad previously. It literally creates space between all the joints of the body, including those between the vertebrae, which relieves pressure on the discs and protects the spine. As your weight increases during pregnancy, you need to guard against a tendency to sag. The extra weight need not pull you down; when it is carried correctly, you can continue to grow and become light.

Paying attention to Tadasana also helps you to understand the other asanas, since the principles of posture are always the same.

## Trikonasana, Triangle Pose

This is a beautiful and simple posture which can be practised right to the end of pregnancy. It develops the feet and legs, encouraging the feeling of being well-grounded, and stretches the spine and the whole trunk so that plenty of space is made for the baby. This lovely stretch can be obtained right up to the day of birth without any strain, especially if a low support is used as shown on the right of the photograph (see Fig. 3.5). To do Trikonasana properly, especially important during pregnancy, it is essential not to bend at the waist, shortening and crumpling the lower side of the trunk. The lower side, from hip to armpit, should extend out from the top of the thigh, so that the upper side of the trunk flattens and extends in parallel fashion. The movement has to come from the hips.

To practise Trikonasana, start by standing with your feet parallel, about three feet apart (or the length of one of your own legs apart). Turn your left foot inwards slightly towards the right and turn the right foot out 90 degrees, keeping the heel of the right foot in line with the centre of the left instep. The whole of the right leg should turn outwards from the hip joint so that the front of the thigh and the kneecap face in the same direction as the toes. At the same time, turn your left thigh outwards as much as possible (it will probably tend to roll in towards the right), lift the arch of the left foot and the inner ankle, and keep the weight firmly on the outer edge of the foot.

Raise your arms to shoulder level so that they are parallel to the floor, with your palms facing down. Relax your shoulders down as you stretch your arms from shoulder to fingertips. With an exhalation, move both your hips to the left and stretch out to the right, making as much space as possible between the right hip and the right armpit. When you have stretched your right ribs out and down as far as you can, place your right hand either on the ground behind your right foot, or on

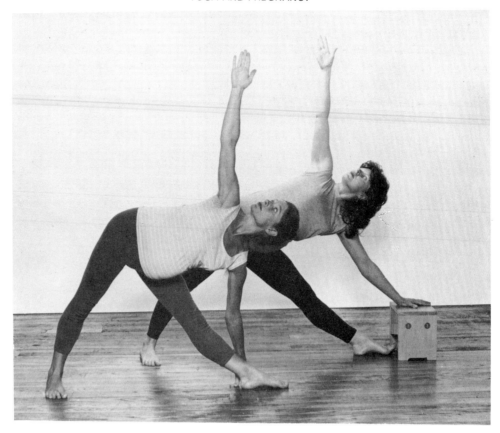

**3.5** Trikonasana

your right ankle or shin, or on a box, stool, chair or other support. You should place your hand on the floor or ankle only if you can do so without bending at the waist. Place the lower hand down very lightly, without taking any weight on it; keep your weight firmly in the legs. If you press your feet into the ground, especially the back foot, you will be able to extend the lumbar spine well, making more space for the baby. Your upper arm should stretch vertically up, palm facing forward, in line with the lower arm. Keep your neck lengthening away from your shoulders towards the crown of your head, in line with the rest of the spine. If it puts strain on your neck to look up at the outstretched hand, then simply look straight ahead of you, keeping your chin in.

Hold the asana for as long as is comfortable with normal breathing. To come up, move both hips back towards the right and stand up in one smooth movement from the centre of the body; this should be done on an inhalation. Repeat the pose to the left, reversing the directions.

## Virabhadrasana II, Second Warrior Pose

This is another posture that can be practised right up to the end of pregnancy.

22

Although it looks simple, for many people it is difficult to do well, for it can be hard to tell whether one is properly centred. It is important that both sides of the trunk should stretch up evenly, as if in Tadasana, without disturbing the posture by leaning to the left or to the right. It is also important, as in all the standing poses, and especially during pregnancy, to lengthen the lumbar spine, avoiding the hollow back, creating space in the trunk and toning the abdominal muscles.

To practise Virabhadrasana II (see Fig. 3.6), stand with your feet about four feet

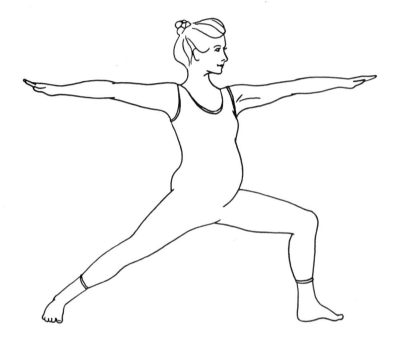

**3.6**   Virabhadrasana II

apart, or just wider than the length of your own leg. Start with your feet parallel, then turn them as described for Trikonasana, so that your left foot turns inwards and your right leg and foot turn out 90 degrees, keeping the right heel exactly in line with the centre of the left inner arch. Raise your arms to shoulder level without lifting your shoulders. Keep plenty of space between your ears and shoulders and let your shoulder blades widen apart from each other. Make sure that your arms are really stretching from shoulder to fingertips, so that you feel the skin coming to life all the way along, without tensing the wrists or the hands. Hands, wrists and fingers should be neither floppy nor rigid.

With an exhalation, bend your right knee by moving your buttock bones down towards the floor, until your knee is immediately above the right ankle. The shin bone should be perpendicular. You must pay careful attention to the pelvis and lower spine; keep the coccyx (tail-bone) moving downwards, without letting the right knee or the left thigh roll forwards; this means that you must become wide

23

across the hip bones in the front as well as the back. As the pelvis widens, the lumbar spine can lengthen upwards, again creating space for the baby and avoiding strain on the lower back. Let any tension in the shoulders and upper body drop down towards your centre of gravity in the pelvis, so that you feel both stable and light, with the spine seeming to grow upwards rather than being held up.

Hold the asana, breathing normally, then rest with your arms relaxed before repeating it, this time to the left.

To check that your back is straight, try practising Virabhadrasana II in front of a mirror. To practise the 'opening' of the hips, you could do the posture using a wall or a piece of heavy furniture as support. Instead of raising your arms, place your hands on your hips and thighs to feel how they are stretching. Use the support behind you as a guide to the correct position of your legs and back; keep the bent knee pressed back against it, rotate the inner thigh of the straight leg away from it, keep the tail-bone moving down it, and bring your lumbar spine towards it. Even better than a wall is a long pole, held for you by a friend, as shown for Tadasana (see Fig. 3.4).

### Uttihita Parsvakonasana

When done correctly, this posture feels marvellous whatever stage of pregnancy you have reached. It is a continuation of the previous posture, Virabhadrasana II, and some women may find it more comfortable than Virabhadrasana, as the weight of the baby on the pelvis is lessened by the sideways position of the trunk. Parsvakonasana enlivens the whole body, creating a powerful stretch along each side in turn, lengthening the spine, opening the hips and stretching the inner thighs. In the later months of pregnancy, you may find the pose more comfortable if you rest your hand on a low support rather than on the floor, as demonstrated on the left of the picture (see Fig. 3.7). Beginners should not place the hand on the floor.

To practise Parsvakonasana, start from Virabhadrasana, as described above. From this position, reach out sideways as far as you can, elongating the lower side of the trunk from hip to armpit, and place your hand lightly on the ground in front of the right foot, or on a block or low stool behind it. You should be trying to close the space between the lower right ribs and the right thigh; if this is not possible, you should definitely have a support under the right hand, otherwise you will distort the posture in your attempt to reach the floor. The whole of the back of the body, from the back of the left heel, through the buttocks and spine, to the shoulders and upper arm, should be in one plane. To begin with, stretch your upper arm up vertically, as shown in the figure behind; then, if you are able, extend your arm alongside your right ear, palm facing down. Hold the posture with normal breathing. Turn your head on its axis to look up in front of your outstretched arm, or simply look straight ahead with your chin in and the back of your neck continuing the line of your spine. Hold the pose for as long as it feels invigorating, not so long that you feel exhausted.

While holding Parsvakonasana, work on the hips and legs as described in the

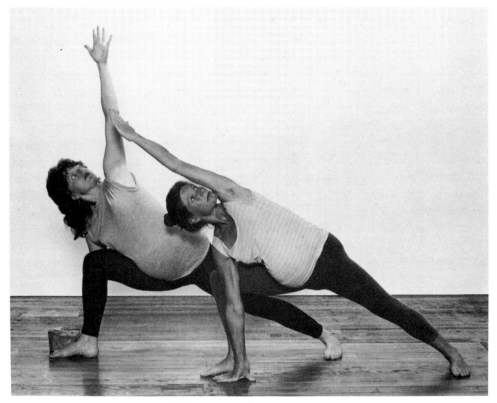

**3.7** Uttihita Parsvakonasana

instructions for Virabhadrasana II. If you have your lower hand on the ground in front of the foot, you can use the arm to help press the bent knee back so that it stays in line with the ankle joint. At the same time try to move the right hip forward and continue to rotate the left hip and thigh outwards to 'open' the hips across the front as well as the back. Press the outer left foot firmly into the ground, lifting the inner arch and ankle, and let the lumbar spine elongate and release out of the pelvis.

When coming out of this pose, inhale as you straighten the right leg and stand up, keeping your weight in the heels. Rest for a few moments before repeating the pose on the other side, to the left.

## Virabhadrasana I, First Warrior Pose

This is a strong, jubilant posture, the kind of pose one practises spontaneously when full of joie de vivre. Practising it regularly will develop your sense of energy and power – it is a good, positive pose for pregnant women to do! Do not be afraid to stretch your arms up; it helps to gain the feeling of stretch and lightness in the upper body, and also creates space in the abdomen, relieving pressure on the uterus and the baby. In the photograph (see Fig. 3.8), the figure on the left is

25

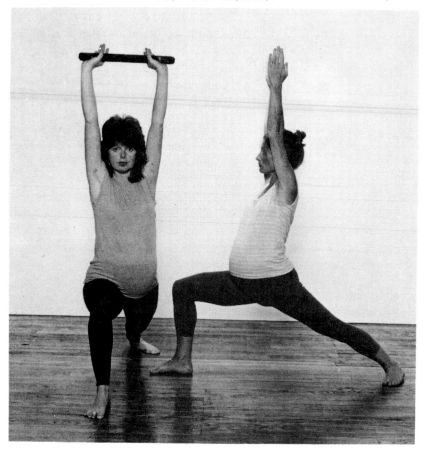

**3.8** Virabhadrasana I

holding a heavy metal bar to encourage this stretch by providing resistance to push against. However, sometimes stretching the arms up can make you feel dizzy, especially at the beginning or end of pregnancy. If this is the case, you can practise this posture without raising your arms, placing your hands on your hips instead. Avoid raising the arms in this pose if you have high blood pressure.

To practise Virabhadrasana I, start by standing with your feet the same distance apart as for the previous two postures, feet parallel. After raising your arms to shoulder level, turn your palms up and stretch your arms straight up above your head. Concentrate on straightening the elbows and bringing the upper arms close together and back, behind the ears if possible. Keep your breathing relaxed. Turn your whole body to the right, turning hips, navel, ribs and chest, until it is facing the same direction as the right foot and knee. Now bend your right knee, with an exhalation, until the shin bone is vertical and the knee directly above the ankle, keeping the left leg straight, the outer left foot pressing down to the floor and the inner arch lifting. As you bend the knee, and while you hold the pose, move the coccyx (tail-bone) downwards, so that you can take any excessive curve out of the

26

small of the back, lengthening the lumbar spine upwards. This is very important; if you do not work on the tail bone, the lumbar will hollow, a position of weakness and strain, especially during pregnancy, and the stomach muscles will sag. As you lengthen your lower back, the front of your body should also lift up out of the pelvis, creating more space between the top of the right thigh and the navel. Keep your face and throat relaxed, and hold the pose for as long as you like without feeling strain.

Inhale as you straighten the right leg, relax your arms and rest for a moment before repeating to the left.

## Forward bending postures

### *Relaxed Uttanasana, Standing Forward Bend*

Uttanasana is a good resting pose to do after the more strenuous standing postures. It rests the upper body, including the heart, and allows blood to circulate freely in the trunk and head. It is a useful pose for relieving tension in the neck and shoulders.

The photographs (see Figs 3.9 and 3.10) show Uttanasana done in the ninth month of pregnancy. For some women, this posture will be comfortable until then,

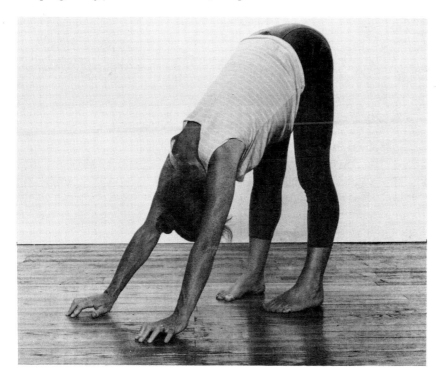

**3.9**  Uttanasana, stage 1

27

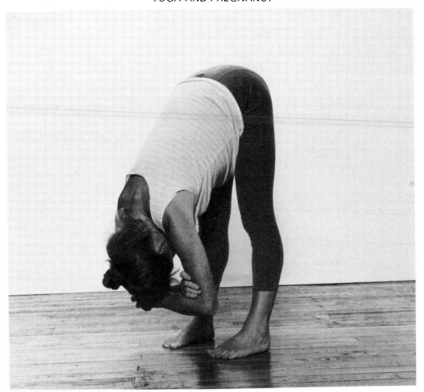

**3.10** Uttanasana, relaxed

for others, it may have to be discontinued halfway through the pregnancy. It depends on how well you are able to lift the buttock bones and widen the pelvis, so that you are truly bending from the hips and not from the waist, or any other part of the spine. If the spine can elongate from the hips, the front of the body will lengthen and open also, and the abdomen will not feel squashed. Do not practise Uttanasana without first doing the spine stretches described on p. 15, and only proceed with Uttanasana if you can do these stretches with a straight back. If you reach the stage where Uttanasana is no longer comfortable, you can rest between the standing poses by bending forward on to a chair (see Fig. 3.2).

To practise Uttanasana, stand with your feet parallel, hip width apart. Place your hands on your hips so that you can feel the movement of the pelvis, and with an exhalation stretch forward from the hips, keeping your back straight and lifting and widening the buttock bones as you bend. When your back is horizontal, with one or both hands lift the lower abdomen forward, freeing it from the top of the thighs. In this way you make plenty of space in the front of the body and the uterus will not be squashed (this becomes necessary some time after the fourth month). Now continue bending from the hips, stretching your arms out in front of you along the floor (see Fig. 3.9).

Plant your heels firmly into the ground and lift the buttock bones higher and higher, releasing into the stretch in the back of the thighs. Widen the buttock bones so that the spine can free itself from the pelvis; imagine that you are literally making space for the spine to unwedge itself and move forward. When you have allowed the spine to elongate as much as possible, relax your arms and just let them hang down towards the floor, or hold your upper arms just above the elbows (see Fig. 3.10). Either way, let the shoulders, arms and entire upper body relax completely. Pay special attention to your neck, face and throat, letting all tension drop away from you to the ground.

Hold the position for as long as you like, providing that your abdomen does not feel squashed, your back does not hurt, and breathing is not difficult. When you stand up, lift your head first and, inhaling, unbend from the hips with a straight back.

## Parsvottanasana

This posture is extremely valuable during pregnancy and afterwards, not only for the way in which it stretches the legs and spine, but also because it opens the chest and frees the shoulders and upper back. This area can become very stiff and tense, starting in pregnancy with the increased weight of the breasts and a tendency to be pulled forward generally by the extra weight of the growing baby. Then, after the birth, the many hours spent feeding and carrying the baby (especially if in a sling on the front of the body) can result in a hunched posture and a great deal of tension in the neck, shoulders and upper back.

I have broken the practice of Parsvottanasana into stages. In *stage 1*, use a chair to help you. Stand with your feet about three feet apart, as for Trikonasana, with the chair placed a short distance away from you on your right. Place

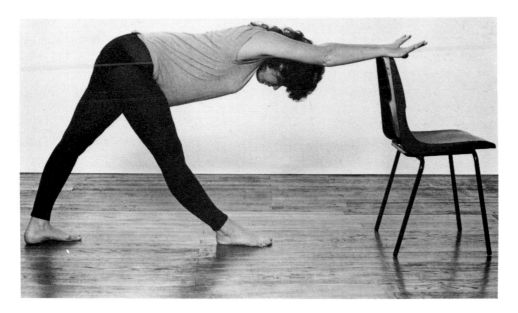

your hands on your hips and then turn your feet and your whole body to the right, so that you are facing the chair. Your right foot and kneecap, the front of your right thigh and both your hips should be directly facing the chair. Your left foot should be turned well in towards the right so that your hips are able to turn properly, and the outer edge of the left heel and the little toe should stay firmly on the floor. By keeping your hands on your hips you can feel whether they are in the right position; the left hip should move forward until it is in line with the right hip. Do not let either hip bone drop down; in other words, keep the pelvis level, and stretch up through the whole body, as in Tadasana.

With an exhalation, stretch towards the back of the chair, hinging at the hips, and reaching out with your arms so that your hands rest lightly on it (Fig. 3.11). Look at the floor so that the back of your neck continues the horizontal line of the spine. Breathe normally, and on every exhalation let the spine release forward a little more; it should be quite flat. All the time keep your feet alive, your legs straight, and concentrate on lifting the buttock bones and drawing them back, away from your head. Try to keep your back, shoulders, neck and arms parallel to the ground. The stretch in the back of the right leg is quite intense, so it is necessary to concentrate on releasing and lengthening the back of the thigh, so that the buttock bones can lift and stay level with each other.

When you have had a good stretch with your right leg forward, inhale as you stand up, and then repeat the pose to the left.

Once you are used to practising this pose with the help of a chair, you can move on to *stage 2*: discard the chair and keep the palms of the hands joined behind your back. Stand with your feet hip width apart while you place your hands together behind your back, with *fingers pointing downwards*. Then turn your wrists so that your fingers point in towards your spine, and continue turning until they point upwards as shown in the picture (see Fig. 3.12). Bring your hands as high as you can without lifting your shoulders. Drop your shoulders down and back, and press your elbows as far back as possible, joining your hands properly so that the index fingers and thumbs move together.

If this position is difficult for you, practise it several times a day at odd moments until your shoulders start to loosen. It is well worth persevering with it because it is such a valuable exercise for improving posture and breathing. Regular practice can save you a great deal of tension and discomfort, especially after your baby is born.

With your hands behind your back, spread your feet about three feet apart and turn your whole body to the right in exactly the same way as described above for stretching on to the chair. Turn your hips until they are level with each other and stretch your whole body upwards (see Fig. 3.13). Keep your feet alive and well grounded on the floor, lift your ankles, stretch your legs, lift the trunk out of the pelvis and lift the breast-bone. Move down only with the tail-bone and the shoulders. You should have no feeling of strain, only a sense of standing tall and open, a feeling of firmness and lightness, not of rigidity.

Next, without losing this stretch, move into stage 3. Exhale as you bend forward

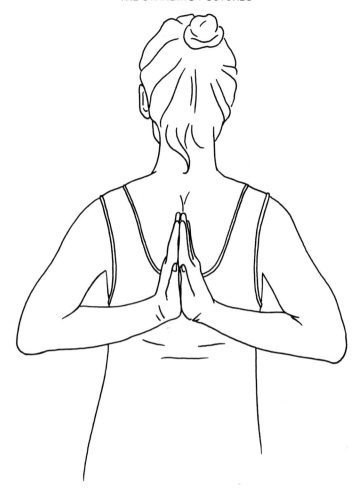

**3.12**  Parsvottanasana, arm position

from the hips in the same way as when reaching out to the chair, but now keeping your palms glued together behind your back and your elbows pressing firmly back like wings (see Fig. 3.14). Look at the floor, keeping your spine horizontal, and breathe normally.

When you stand up, do so on an inhalation, lifting your head first. Repeat the posture on the other side, turning your feet and whole body to the left.

*Note*: The final stage of Parsvottanasana is to continue bending until the chest and then the chin touch the right leg. This can be practised in the early part of pregnancy up to about the fourth month, until the abdomen begins to enlarge, but then it should be discontinued.

### Prasarita Padottanasana

This is a beautiful asana to practise during pregnancy. It is one of the more stable

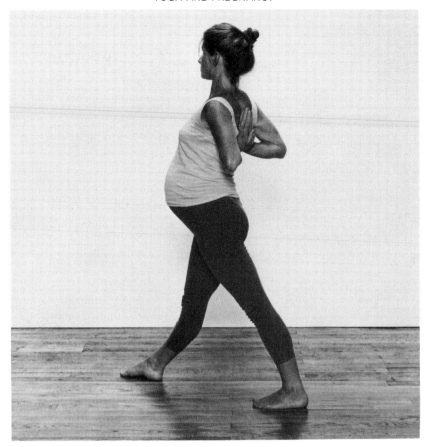

**3.13**  Parsvottanasana, stage 2

poses, with hands and feet planted firmly on the ground. The weight of the uterus is taken off the spine completely and the posture can be held for quite a long time without strain, really enabling the spine to release and lengthen.

To practise Prasarita Padottanasana, stand with your feet spread about four feet apart, wider than for Trikonasana. Keep your feet parallel. The principles of bending forward for this posture are exactly the same as for Uttanasana and Parsvottanasana – the body must hinge in the groin and not in the waist. If you are stiff in the lower back and backs of the legs and find it difficult to rotate the pelvis forward keeping a straight back, then do not attempt to place your hands on the floor straight away. Instead, practise this pose with your hands resting on the back of a chair, then progress to placing your hands on the chair seat. In other words, you will be stretching in the same way as shown in figs. 3.14 and 3.15 (page 33), except that your feet are spread further apart.

When you are able to bend easily from the hips, you can discard the chair and embark on *stage 1*: place your hands on the ground. Put them down so that they divide the space between the feet evenly, and make sure to spread out the palms and the fingers as wide as you can. Have your middle fingers pointing directly

32

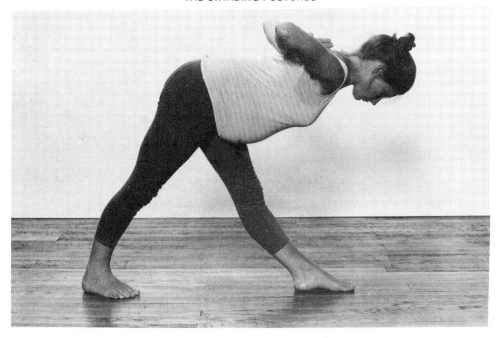

**3.14** Parsvottanasana, stage 3

forwards. Look down at the floor, keeping your neck and the back of your head in line with the rest of the spine, and breathe normally (see Fig. 3.15).

Feel the ground under your feet and hands, experiencing the contact between it and the skin on soles and palms. Keep your toes and fingers stretched and relaxed. Do not lean on your hands, but keep all your weight in the legs. Lift the inner

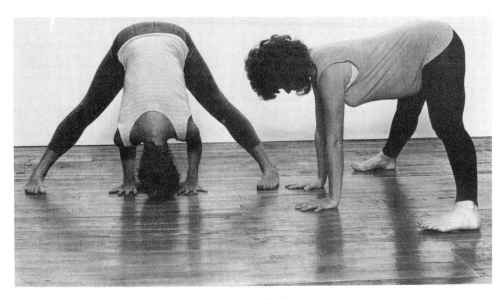

**3.15** Prasarita Padottanasana

33

arches of the feet and the inner ankles. Let the backs of the legs stretch and do not let the knees roll in. If you concentrate on spreading the buttock bones apart, you will find that the spine will stretch forward easily and pleasurably, with a sense of release. Do not hollow the back – this is especially important when you are pregnant.

When you have extended your spine and the front of your body as far forward as possible, you can try *stage 2* (shown on the left, Fig. 3.15): lower the trunk to place your head on or near the floor, with your elbows bent directly backwards. Try this position only if you can keep the front of the body really well extended from groin to breast-bone, so that you do not lose the space you have made for the baby in the first part of the exercise. It helps if you think in terms of moving your breast-bone to the floor rather than your head; your spine should remain as straight as possible. There is no benefit in practising this stage if you feel the front of your body folding and becoming squashed. You will feel when and if it is wise to discontinue this position as your pregnancy progresses.

To come up, lift your head and straighten your arms on an inhalation. Then place your hands on your hips and inhale again as you stand up. Bring your feet together gently.

## Postures which develop balance

### Parivrtta Trikonasana, Reverse Triangle Pose

Parivrtta Trikonasana is the only reversed standing posture that can be done after the fourth month of pregnancy and is valuable for the way in which it helps prevent and relieve backache. Parsvottanasana (p. 29) is a good preparation for this pose.

This is not strictly a balancing pose in the sense of standing on one leg, but it does require and develop good balance because of the way the hips are turned and the narrow plane in which the body is aligned. In the second part of pregnancy, balance is helped by placing the lower hand on a stool rather than on the floor, as illustrated here (see Fig. 3.16). This also raises the trunk, opening the front of the body more and making space for the enlarging uterus.

To practise Parivrtta Trikonasana, start by moving into stage 1 of Parsvottanasana, as illustrated on p. 29, Fig. 3.11, and have a low support such as a stool by your right foot. Then, exhaling, turn your hips and trunk further to the right, placing your left hand on the stool and stretching your right arm vertically up, the palm of the right hand facing in the same direction as your chest. As you turn the hips, make sure that your left foot stays firmly on the ground, with the outer heel and little toe making contact with the floor. Lift the inner arches of both feet, lift the inner ankles, and do not let the feet roll inwards. Keep your knees straight and let the backs of the legs stretch from heels to buttock bones, turning the hips as much as you can. In this pose, unlike Parsvottanasana, the right hip is slightly higher than the left. Drawing your right hip back and pressing your left

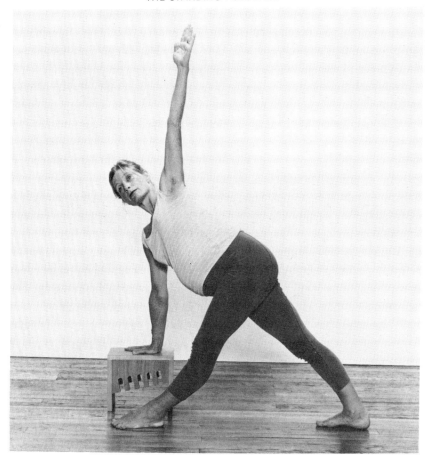

**3.16** Parivrtta Trikonasana

foot firmly on to the ground will help you to extend the lumbar spine. Do not lean your weight into the hand which is resting on the stool.

Breathe normally while you hold the posture, then inhale as you stand up straight, swinging up from the hips, and repeat the pose to the left.

### Vrksasana, Tree Pose

This posture can give you a beautiful stretch during pregnancy, but it is not really recommended if you are a complete beginner, since it takes some practice before the hips become open and stable enough for the trunk to lift up evenly from them. If the posture is collapsed or crooked, there is no benefit for you or the baby. However, if in doubt you can try Vrksasana with your back against a wall to help you to balance, and to find out whether it feels good. If you are not used to balancing on one leg, practise the leg stretching exercise illustrated on p. 14, Fig. 3.1.

To practise Vrksasana, begin in Tadasana. Transfer your weight to your right foot and pick up your left ankle with your hands and place the left foot against the inner right thigh, toes pointing downwards (see Fig. 3.17). Press your heel in firmly and do not grip with the toes. Keep your right leg firm and straight, with your weight balanced evenly on the right foot. Move your tail-bone down and press your bent left knee back to widen the hips. Stretch up well from the tops of the legs so that neither hip collapses, and keep plenty of space between the pelvis and the lower ribs.

Stretch your arms above your head as shown, keeping the upper arms close to

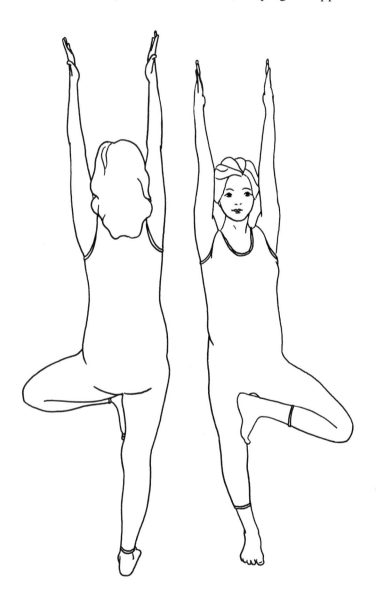

**3.17** Vrksasana

the head, and maintaining space between shoulders and ears. Do not tense your wrists or hands. Try to stretch both sides of the body up evenly; you should be standing as you would in Tadasana except that you are on one leg and your arms are raised. If your balance is uncertain, practise next to a wall.

Lower your arms, stand evenly on both feet again, and re-align yourself in Tadasana before repeating the pose on the other leg.

### Ardha Chandrasana, Half Moon Pose or Triangle Balance

This posture creates a wonderful feeling of space and lightness in the body. When practised against a wall as illustrated (see Fig. 3.18), it is not strenuous; it can be held for some time and can be done until the end of pregnancy. However, you need to start practising it in early pregnancy to become used to moving into it correctly before your weight increases very much; otherwise you will find it hard to get into position without help. Like the other balancing postures, this pose will not come well unless the feet and ankles are strong and supple. For these reasons, it is not usually suitable for beginners.

To practise Ardha Chandrasana, stand with your back against a wall with your

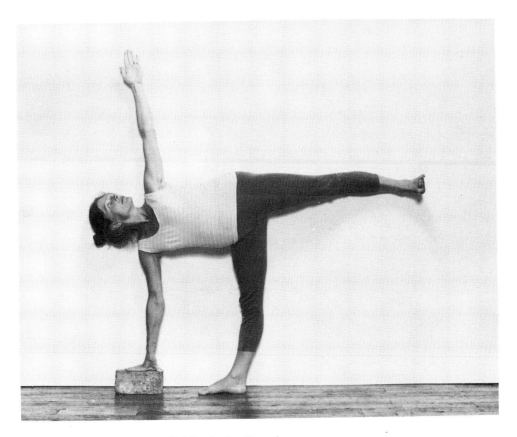

**3.18** Ardha Chandrasana

37

feet about three feet apart, as for Trikonasana. Put a brick or a pile of books by the wall to your right. Prepare to do Trikonasana to the right, with the brick about nine inches away from your out-turned right foot. Keep your right foot exactly parallel to the wall and the right heel in line with the centre of the left instep. With an exhalation, move into Trikonasana (see p. 22). Hold Trikonasana with normal breathing and stretch your spine to its maximum before proceeding. Also ground your feet well, lifting the arches, and spreading the toes, and rotate both thighs outwards as much as possible.

Now, without losing this action in the thighs, bend your right knee and take your weight on to your right foot, lifting your left foot slightly from the floor. At the same time, reach out with your right hand and rest it on the brick. With an exhalation, straighten your right leg, lifting your left leg up the wall, heel touching the wall, toes pointing forwards. Your left leg and trunk should now be horizontal. Keep your shoulders and back of your hips turned back against the wall and spread out the toes of your left foot. Stretch your left arm up vertically in line with the right arm, with the palm of the hand facing forward, as in Trikonasana. Breathe normally.

Do not lean your weight against the wall, or into your right hand. Use the wall for balance and alignment, but keep your weight entirely in the right leg. This supporting leg should feel as though it is growing longer, stretching up to the right hip, the right thigh rotating back towards the wall. The left thigh must also rotate back, so helping to open the hips, bringing the left hip closer to the wall. The raised left leg and the trunk should stretch out, with even energy, horizontally away from each other. The shoulders should widen and move away from the ears, allowing the neck to extend towards the crown of the head. You can either look straight ahead, keeping your chin in and the back of your neck against the wall, or you can turn your head on its axis and look at the upper hand, as shown in the photograph.

To come out of this pose, bend your right knee and carefully lower your left foot to the floor. Now straighten your right leg so that you return to Trikonasana and inhale as you stand up, swinging the trunk up from the hips. Repeat the posture to the left.

*Chapter 4*

# The Sitting Postures

'The practice of yoga generally helped me keep in touch with my body when it was going through so many changes. I found the standing poses were very good for my balance, circulation, digestion and for strengthening my back. I found the sitting poses, those where your legs are open, very good for opening the pelvis. I found it marvellous just sitting in a pose, the baby would start kicking and I used to sit there and talk to him! I felt that he was enjoying it too! I particularly liked to lie on my back with my legs up the wall – I found that really good for resting the legs.'

*Amanda*

Included in this section are the sitting or kneeling postures that are most useful and enjoyable in pregnancy, especially late pregnancy. In the first four months, the whole range of forward bends, twists and back bends can be done as usual, and the more experienced student may be able to continue most of them for longer than that; it is a question of what feels right for each individual woman. However, if you are a beginner in yoga, the basic postures shown in this book are the ones you can do throughout the nine months, and are, in any case, the ones which are most valuable in pregnancy. They stretch the legs and spine, strengthen the back and teach one how to sit well at all times in everyday life, whether on a chair or on the floor. They also increase flexibility in the ankle, knee and hip joints. This means that if you are stiff when you first become pregnant, regular practice of the basic sitting postures will soon enable you to adopt positions that are beneficial to you and the baby as the pregnancy progresses. For example, sitting cross-legged or kneeling on a firm surface is better for your spine, and makes more space for the baby, than leaning back in a soft armchair; and once your joints become more supple, you will find sitting in this way much more comfortable anyway.

As for the birth itself, the way in which the sitting postures affect the pelvic area will increase the chances of an enjoyable and straightforward labour. The asanas in the middle part of this section are especially valuable, which is why they have been classified as 'essential pregnancy postures'. They stretch the inner thighs, which can be tight and resistant, and also open the hips. They improve circulation to the whole pelvic area, and will make you aware of the muscles around the pelvis and in the pelvic floor, so you can learn to release them through concentration and deep breathing. This is clearly of great importance during labour, when any

39

tension here can seriously obstruct the normal process of birth. The pelvic area is one in which old fears and emotional tensions can become locked in tight muscles; tight hips and thighs are really quite common, and working carefully on this area of the body can produce a great sense of relief and freedom. The actual process of releasing the hips and thighs into the stretch is a valuable preparation for relaxing during the contractions of labour. In both cases, you have to have trust in your body before you are able to let go.

The best way to approach the sitting postures is to allow a little time each day for working on one or two of them with complete concentration (especially those you find most difficult), so that you can discover exactly where your own 'blocks' are and how to release them with the help of the breath. In addition, you can practise sitting and kneeling in any of these positions at other times in the day while you are doing something else, such as talking to friends, reading, working with your hands, playing with children, etc. You will soon come to prefer sitting on the floor to sitting on chairs. When you do have to sit on a chair, you can keep your postural awareness by sitting well forward on your buttock bones, so that the spine does not collapse backwards. This is easiest on a hard chair, but can still be done on a soft chair if you tuck your feet under you and sit cross-legged.

## Basic sitting and forward bending

### *Dandasana, Staff Pose, Basic Sitting*

As Tadasana is to the standing postures, so Dandasana is to the sitting poses: it is the basic sitting posture and should be practised all the way through pregnancy and after. It keeps the hamstring muscles stretched and strengthens the back. It will teach you how to stretch the spine evenly, from coccyx to neck, neither overworking nor collapsing any part of it; and it brings life and alertness to the whole person.

In the standard pose, the hands are placed lightly on the ground beside the hips, and those who have the strength and suppleness to maintain this position without strain can do so throughout pregnancy. Figure 4.1 shows alternative ways of obtaining a good position when a little support is desired. In the background, a rolled blanket is placed under the buttocks to ensure that the pelvis is not rotating backwards with the weight falling on to the coccyx; this lift under the buttocks is essential for those with tight hamstrings or a very stiff lower back. The weight should be taken on the front part of the buttock bones, with the pelvis vertical and the spine able to stretch up evenly. It is very important to get the base of the posture right, otherwise there will be strain in the back. If in doubt, always use the blanket, or a wedge of the type shown on p. 45.

The upturned chair is used in two ways. The feet can be placed against the bottom of the seat, thus keeping them even and keeping all the toes in line. In Dandasana, the little toes and big toes should be the same distance away from the

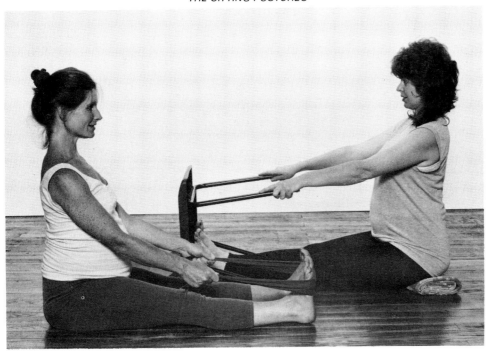

**4.1** Dandasana

head. If there is a tendency for the big toes to come forward, it means that the inner legs are not stretching enough, and the chair should be used to correct this. The legs of the chair are used to hold on to in order to help straighten the legs and the back. In the foreground, a belt is held around the feet to the same effect.

To practise Dandasana, sit either on the floor or on the front edge of a firmly rolled blanket. Have your chair or belt near you. With your hands take hold of the flesh of the buttocks and pull it back and sideways so that you can feel the points of the buttock bones making contact with the ground. Now pull your chair towards you, or loop your belt around your feet, and stretch both legs firmly away from you, making sure that all the toes are the same distance away and that the backs of the knees are pressing towards the floor. As your bulge gets bigger, you will find it more comfortable to keep your legs slightly apart. Holding lightly on to the chair legs or the ends of the belt, feel your way into letting your spine stretch up, and with it the front of the body, by grounding the buttock bones firmly and lifting and widening the pelvis (just as you do when stretching the spine forward from the standing position, as shown on p. 15.

Beware of trying to *pull* yourself up and creating tension in your upper back and arms; make sure that your shoulders stay down and relaxed and use your hands and arms to bring more awareness into your back. You should feel light and free in the upper body as the spine grows out of the pelvis and as the ribs and breast-bone lift, making more space for the baby.

41

Hold the position with normal or deep breathing for as long as is comfortable, and if you wish, proceed with the following posture, Paschimottanasana.

## Paschimottanasana, Sitting Forward Bend

This posture, a continuation of Dandasana, should be done only by those who are loose enough in the hamstring muscles for the pelvis to be able to rotate forward with straight legs, so that the bending movement comes entirely from the hips and not from the middle of the back. The back should remain straight. The degree to which you can bend forward is obviously determined by the size of the abdomen. In the first half of pregnancy, you may be able to hold your toes; later you will have to use the belt or the chair.

To practise Paschimottanasana, first sit in Dandasana. If using the chair, make sure that your feet are flat against the seat of the chair; if using the belt, place it around the balls of the feet so as to stretch the backs of the legs really well. Spread your toes and stretch your legs out and your spine up as much as you can, sitting well forward on your buttock bones (see Fig. 4.2). Before rotating the pelvis forward (or as you do so), you can lift the abdomen forward with one or both hands so as to lift the uterus clear of the thighs and stop it from getting squashed (see Uttanasana, p. 28).

Then, with an exhalation, stretch forward by rotating the pelvis in such a way that the front hip bones lift and move forward at the same time. Do not let the front hip bones collapse downwards, otherwise the baby is squashed. Keep your buttock

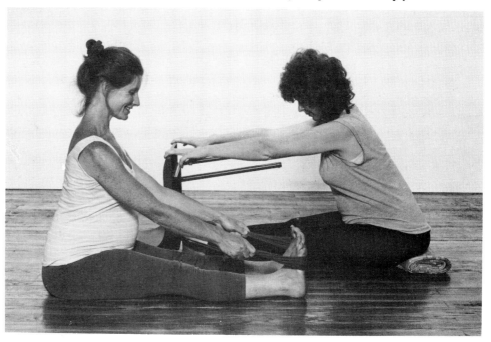

**4.2** Paschimottanasana

bones firmly on the ground and feel the space between them widening, as for Uttanasana, the standing forward bend. The lumbar spine should be extending, not becoming convex, and the front of the body should continue to feel open and free as in Dandasana. Bend only as far as the size of your abdomen allows – this will be further if you spread your legs slightly wider apart. If using the chair, you can stretch your hands towards the chair seat as you bend forwards; if using the belt, gather it up in your hands as you reach nearer to your feet. Breathe normally. Keep your neck and the back of your head aligned with your back, chin in, as shown, with your face looking forward.

neck and the back of your head aligned with your back, chin in, as shown, with your feet looking forward.

Hold the posture for as long as is comfortable, then inhale as you return to Dandasana.

*Note*: if you normally practise Paschimottanasana in its completed form, with your head resting on your knees or shins, then you can continue with this until the fourth month of pregnancy, or until the abdomen begins to enlarge noticeably. Thereafter modify the pose gradually as you grow bigger.

## Janu Sirsasana, Head to Knee Pose

This forward-bending posture feels comfortable during pregnancy because the angle made between the two thighs leaves plenty of room for the large abdomen. In the completed form of Janu Sirsasana, as in Paschimottanasana, the head is placed on the knee or shin of the outstretched leg. However, after about the fourth month this is no longer comfortable, so the posture is done bending forward no more than half way, keeping the back straight.

To practise Janu Sirsasana, start in Dandasana with your belt within reach. Bend your left leg, placing the sole of your left foot near the inner right thigh, if possible slightly away from it (see Fig. 4.3). Draw your left heel back as near to the groin as possible, keeping the bent knee relaxed near the ground. Keep your right leg absolutely straight, undisturbed by the change of position of the left leg, with the right kneecap and toes facing upwards, the heel extended firmly away from you.

Now turn your trunk somewhat to the right, in order to bring your breast-bone and navel in line with the centre of your right leg. If you place your left hand on your left knee and your right hand on the ground beside your right hip, this will help you to turn more easily. Now take hold of your right foot by the toes, bending forward from the hips in exactly the same way as for Paschimottanasana. Hold the toes lightly. If you cannot reach the toes easily, then take your belt and loop it around the ball of the right foot, holding the ends of the belt as illustrated. Do not tense your arms or shoulders; simply use the grip on the belt or the foot to help your legs and your spine stretch to their maximum. Stretch your legs actively, the right leg extending firmly away from you, toes spread, and the left knee moving back. Keep the back of your neck and head in line with your spine, chin in.

Inhale as you sit upright, then repeat the posture on the other side (left leg bent).

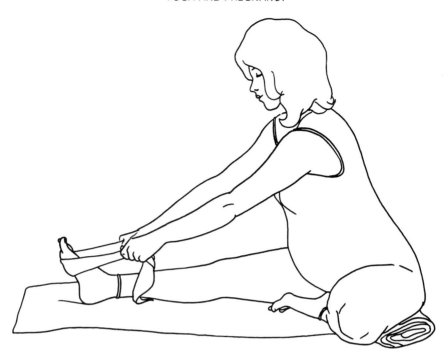

**4.3** Janu Sirsasana

## Essential pregnancy postures

The postures in this group are especially relevant for pregnancy and birth because of the way in which they stretch and tone the muscles of the pelvic floor, helping to make them more effective as a support for the pelvic organs. They also improve circulation, reducing congestion from the weight of the uterus on the pelvic blood vessels. All the postures can be used during labour if they have been practised enough beforehand to be comfortable. They loosen the hip joints and the inner thigh muscles which in many people are tight, and being able to release in these areas requires careful listening to your body; concentration on the breath helps to accept the stretching that takes place. For this reason, these postures are especially suitable as a preparation for breathing through labour contractions. At least two or three of these postures should be done every day during pregnancy. (See note, pp. 90–1.)

### *Baddha Konasana, Cobbler Pose, and variations*

This is a very rewarding posture to practise during pregnancy, and many women find it a comfortable way of sitting during labour. Although most people have difficulty in letting the knees drop to the floor, the pregnancy hormones, which soften the ligaments and tissues, make it easier than usual. If you have had

44

difficulty with the pose previously, you may find that you make rapid progress with it while you are pregnant. As with all the sitting postures, it is important to keep the pelvis vertical so that the spine can stretch up from its base, rather than letting it tilt back so that the weight falls on the coccyx. To this end, place a firmly rolled blanket under the back of the buttock bones, or sit on a specially made wedge, as shown in Fig. 4.4.

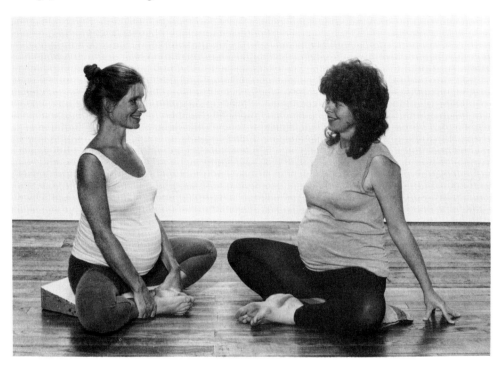

**4.4** Baddha Konasana

To practise Baddha Konasana, sit on your blanket or wedge with the soles of your feet together, as near to the body as possible. With your hands, separate your buttocks so that you settle on the forward part of the buttock bones. An advantage of sitting on a hard surface rather than a soft blanket is that you can clearly feel the contact between it and the buttock bones. If you are not sitting correctly, in other words if you are rolling on to the base of the spine, you will feel strain in the back as you try to maintain the posture, or you will collapse into a hunched back position in which breathing is difficult and the uterus squashed. When you are sitting correctly the posture feels comfortable and stable, breathing can be deep and regular, with the chest open and the breast-bone lifting, and with the head and neck lengthening away from the shoulders. Clasp your toes or ankles and use the grip to help you lift the spine. Alternatively, place your fingertips on the floor behind you and use the pressure of the fingers against the ground to help you to stretch up.

If you practise Baddha Konasana with the support of a wall (see Fig. 4.5), you may find it easier to concentrate on releasing your hips and inner thighs. Sit with your back against the wall and the back of the buttock bones touching the wall. Place your hands on your knees or on your thighs, and stretch up so that you can feel the spine 'growing' up the wall, with only a small space between it and the lumbar area. Let your shoulders relax down and back, so that the top of your chest lifts and the lower points of your shoulder blades move down the wall.

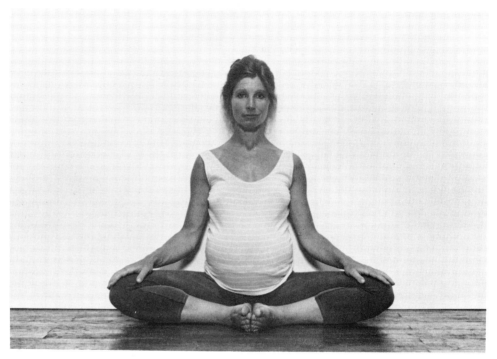

**4.5**   Baddha Konasana, supported

Let your breathing settle into a steady rhythm, then, on every exhalation, concentrate on letting your hips open and your thigh muscles release, so that your knees can drop nearer to the floor. After a few breaths, you can use your hands to press the knees firmly but gently down, exerting pressure only as you exhale, and only if you feel a certain 'give' in the muscles; do not force against resistance, but wait for the resistance to melt with the help of the out-breath. With the support of the wall behind you, you will be able to hold the posture for longer without strain, and you may find that your knees drop dramatically lower without effort or discomfort.

Another variation is to stretch your arms above your head (see Fig. 4.6). This feels wonderful in later pregnancy, because of the way in which it creates space in the whole trunk, relieving any feeling of heaviness from the baby and making breathing easier. (Notice how the bump of the uterus almost disappears in this picture.) Interlock your fingers and extend your arms out in front of you, palms outwards, and keep stretching your arms out as far as possible as you raise them

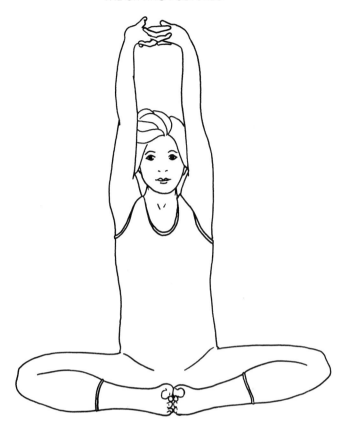

**4.6**  Baddha Konasana, variation

above your head. Do not hollow your back or push your ribs forward; keep the ribs passive and let the spine elongate.

To come out of Baddha Konasana, lift your knees together with your hands, then slide your legs out in front of you along the floor. Come out of the pose gently and slowly, especially if you have been sitting in it for some time.

Baddha Konasana can also be done lying on the floor, to give a completely passive stretch to the hips and legs (see Fig. 4.7). Before lying down, tie your belt firmly round your feet, to keep the soles joined together. Hold the other end of the belt as you lie back so that you can draw your heels closer in towards the body. Let the weight of the legs pull your knees down by force of gravity and consciously relax the places where you feel the stretch.

You can also do this version of Baddha Konasana without the belt, but with your toes against the wall to stop your feet sliding away from you.

When you come out of this position, use your hands to lift your knees up gently.

You can also get a partner to help you in some variations of Baddha Konasana. First, get her to rest her feet on your thighs, as shown in Fig. 4.8, and allow your legs to relax under her weight. A constant, heavy weight helps the muscles to

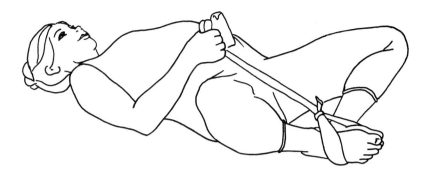

**4.7** Baddha Konasana, variation

release and feels soothing, but never exert pressure in short, jerky movements, as this can cause the muscles to tense and shorten again.

If you are comfortable with the weight on your thighs, get your partner to transfer the weight to your knees, as this will increase the stretch in your thighs and hips.

To take the position a stage further, ask your helper to sit up so that you can reach her shoulders, then clasp your hands around her neck and use the grip to pull

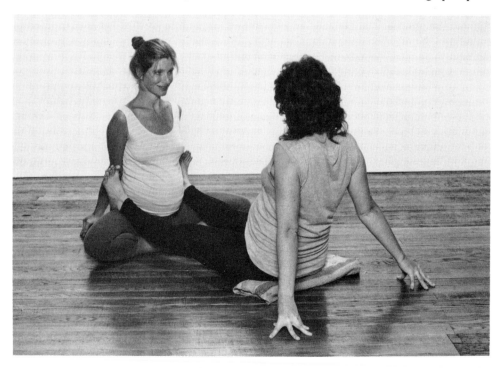

**4.8** Baddha Konasana, variation

yourself up and forward from the pelvis (see Fig. 4.9). When using your arms to help stretch the spine in any of the sitting postures, make sure that you are not simply tensing your hands, arms and shoulders and pulling from the chest. Keep your awareness on the source of the movement, in the pelvis.

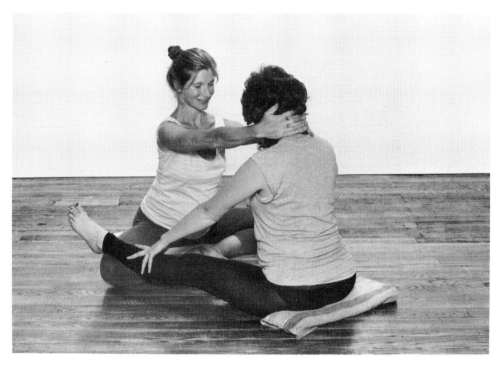

**4.9**   Baddha Konasana, variation

Another variation which is worth trying is shown in Fig. 4.10. This can give a wonderful feeling of freedom and ease. If you tend to collapse the lower back in Baddha Konasana, you will find that the support around your pelvic area takes the strain out of the posture. You need a strong, wide sling, so a length of cloth is better than a belt, which would tend to slide up the back and not give support where it is needed. The weight of your partner's legs not only keeps your knees down, but also stops you from sliding forward as she pulls on the ends of the cloth. If the weight on your knees is too much, she can rest her feet on your thighs instead. The cloth should be looped in a wide band around your lower back, and the direction of pull is forward and up.

When you have held the position for long enough, get your helper to remove her feet gently, to lift your knees together for you, and then pull your feet out along the floor to straighten your legs.

## Upavistha Konasana

This is another posture which is very valuable during pregnancy, and one that

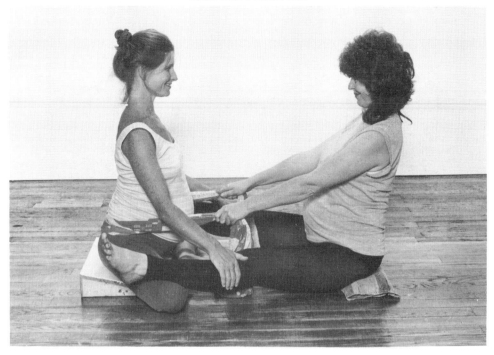

**4.10**   Baddha Konasana, variation

many people normally find difficult due to tightness in the hips, inner thighs and hamstring muscles. It is a posture to approach with patience, because it cannot be forced without risk of injury. However, you may find that you make noticeable progress with this posture during pregnancy because of the loosening effect of the pregnancy hormones. Upavistha Konasana is an excellent posture for adopting often in your everyday life. If you have manual work to do, it can be very comfortable to sit with your legs apart, with a blanket or cushion under the buttocks if needed, and with your work on the floor between your legs. To prevent stiffness from holding the same position for too long, alternate it with Janu Sirsasana (by bending one knee, see Fig. 4.3), and with an easy cross-legged pose.

To practise Upavistha Konasana with a partner, sit facing one another with your legs spread as wide as possible (see Fig. 4.11). Place a wedge or rolled blanket under your hips if your pelvis tilts backwards. Pull the buttock muscles out and back with both hands, so that you are sitting with your weight firmly on your buttock bones. Keep your toes and kneecaps facing upwards, spread your toes and stretch your legs out actively, lengthening the entire back of each leg from hip bone to heel. Clasping each other by the wrists or arms, use this hold to help stretch yourself up out of the hips. Do not tense your arms and shoulders, but use your hands to help feel what is happening in the pelvis and lower spine. Keep your buttock bones and tail-bone moving down into the floor, widen the pelvis and let the spine stretch upwards.

When practising Upavistha Konasana on your own, sit with your hands behind

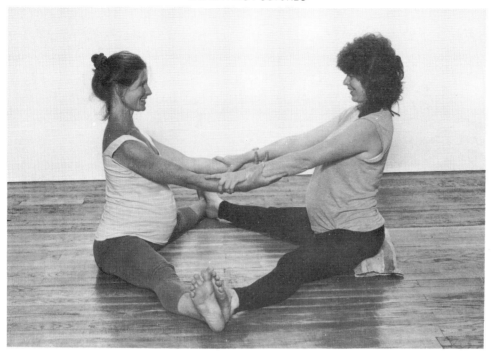

**4.11** Upavistha Konasana

you with your fingertips resting on the floor (see Baddha Konasana, Fig. 4.4). Alternatively, you can sit facing the wall, with your feet against the wall. As you are able to release into the stretch in the legs, you can widen them a little further, moving your hips forward and your feet further apart along the wall.

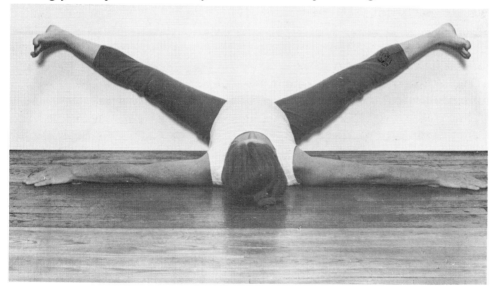

**4.12** Upavistha Konasana, variation

Like Baddha Konasana, this posture can also be done passively, lying on the floor (see Fig. 4.12). Use the wall to support your legs. To get into position, start by sitting sideways against the wall, as close to it as possible. From here, roll on to your back, turning at the same time so that you end up lying on your back with your buttock bones touching the wall and with your feet on the wall, knees bent. Straighten your legs and spread them as wide apart as they will go. Let the weight of your legs pull them down towards the floor by force of gravity. Concentrate on releasing the muscles and hip joints where you feel the pulling sensation, letting go on every exhalation. Stretch the backs of the legs from hip bones to heels, as you do when sitting in Upavistha Konasana. The backs of the knees should be against the wall, the knee caps and toes facing into the centre of the room. You can massage the inner thighs gently to help the muscles to relax.

For a lovely stretch in the upper body, extend your arms behind your head along the floor, but make sure that you do not hollow your back and lift your rib-cage in the attempt to lie your arms on the ground. If your shoulders are stiff, have your arms stretched out to the sides, as shown; and work on your shoulders in the following poses: Virasana (p. 36), Virabhadrasana I (p. 26), Parsvottanasana (p. 29), and Baddha Konasana against the wall (p. 46).

*Note*: some women find in later pregnancy that, if they lie flat on their back, they feel dizzy and uncomfortable. If this happens to you, omit the lying down version of Upavistha Konasana and practise only the sitting posture. Also, very occasionally, women who are normally loose enough in the hips to spread their legs apart with ease, find that during pregnancy, they are over-stretching these joints. This can lead to pain in the lower joints of the back or in the pubic joints at the front of the pelvis. If this is the case, you should avoid Upavistha Konasana and any other sitting posture which loosens the hips and causes the same pain. After the birth, the joints will become more stable again.

## Two Forward Bends

These two positions give a soothing stretch to the spine. They are especially valuable because they allow you to bend forward right up to the end of pregnancy, taking the weight of the baby off the spine and giving some of the benefits of the forward-bending postures that can no longer be practised for fear of squashing the abdomen. Forward-bending postures are calming and relaxing; they quieten the nerves and the mind and have a refreshing effect. It is beneficial for the internal organs to be pulled by gravity away from the spine, relieving compression and improving circulation to them. And, like the other postures in this section, these two poses work on the hip, knee and ankle joints and stretch the thighs.

To practise the cross-legged forward bend, sit on the floor in a comfortable cross-legged position with a chair in front of you (see Fig. 4.13, left). Sit on the buttock bones, separating the flesh with your hands. Make sure you are sitting in a good upright posture before bending forwards, with your weight distributed evenly between the two buttocks and with your spine straight. Bend forward carefully

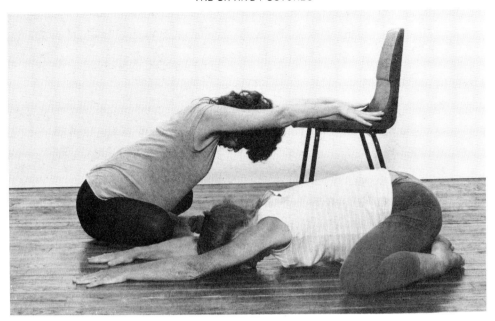

**4.13**   Cross-legged forward bend; kneeling forward bend

from the hips, folding in the groins, and lifting the front hip bones forward and up. Do not collapse any part of the trunk as you stretch forward. Rest your arms and hands on the seat of the chair and hold the position for as long as is comfortable, letting the spine lengthen on every exhalation. Your spine should be flat, not convex. Inhale as you sit up, then repeat the pose with your legs crossed the opposite way round.

To practise the kneeling forward bend or 'Frog' Pose, kneel on the floor, then spread your knees as wide apart as possible and sit on your feet (as shown by the front figure, Fig. 4.13). Your heels should be apart, your toes touching. Bend forward gradually, sliding your arms out along the floor. Relax in this position for as long as you can, releasing tightness in the inner thighs and groins, and letting the spine elongate out of the hips. Do not let the thighs roll in towards each other; pushing the knees outwards relieves pain in the groins and helps the spine to lengthen. Rest your head on the floor so that your neck is relaxed. Ideally, your spine should make a smooth straight line from coccyx to neck. If your spine is very convex, with the vertebrae protruding markedly (look in a mirror, or feel with one hand), then keep your arms bent and rest on your elbows. Alternatively, rest your arms on the seat of a chair as in the previous pose.

When practising this pose in early pregnancy, it is advisable to place a thick folded blanket or cushion on the floor immediately in front of you, so that you can rest your chest against it when you bend forward. If the front of the body can make contact with a firm support, it is easier to relax in the posture and let the spine release.

53

*Squatting*

Squatting forms the basis of several yoga postures and is in itself an extremely valuable position for pregnancy and birth. It is a useful resting pose, easing both backache and heaviness in the pelvic floor due to standing for long periods. In fact, whenever you have to stand, you could squat instead. Squatting also strengthens the feet and ankles and stretches the calf muscles and Achilles tendons, which are often tight. Like the other postures in this section, it improves circulation to the whole pelvic area. It increases your awareness of your pelvic floor muscles, so that you can learn to strengthen and relax them in preparation for birth. And during labour, squatting is a valuable position since it opens the birth canal to its widest, helping the delivery of the baby's head and reducing the likelihood of tearing the perineum.

Along with the other poses in this group, squatting is a position to use as often as possible in your daily life. This is easy in the case of squatting – you can squat every time you want to rest from standing, when you go to the lavatory (if you have a stool to rest your feet on), and when you need to bend down to do something, for example, picking objects up from the floor, taking food from the oven, talking to small children, etc. If you have to lift a child or any heavy object, always squat down to do so, so that you use the strength of your legs to do the lifting and avoid straining your back.

To practise squatting, start by standing with your feet hip width apart and parallel, with a wedge or book placed under your heels (see Fig. 4.14). If you are unsure about your balance, stand near a firm support, such as a table or rail, to hold on to as you bend your knees. Keep your back as long as possible and keep your feet parallel – the tendency is for the toes to turn outwards. Keep your weight distributed evenly between the heels and the balls of the feet, and keep the feet alive, pressing the big toe joints firmly into the floor, lifting the arches, and spreading the toes as you lower yourself into the squatting position. You will probably feel the work going on in the ankles, and a strong stretch in the back of the heels and calves. As this stretch becomes more comfortable and your balance improves, lower the support under the heels. Eventually, you should be able to squat with your feet flat on the floor.

When you stand up from the squatting position, inhale quite deeply and do not come up too quickly, otherwise you may feel dizzy.


## Other useful postures


*Padmasana, Lotus Pose*

Padmasana can be practised throughout pregnancy and brings suppleness to the hip, knee and ankle joints. It is a good, stable sitting posture in which to practise deep breathing or meditation, and in which to have a really good stretch of the

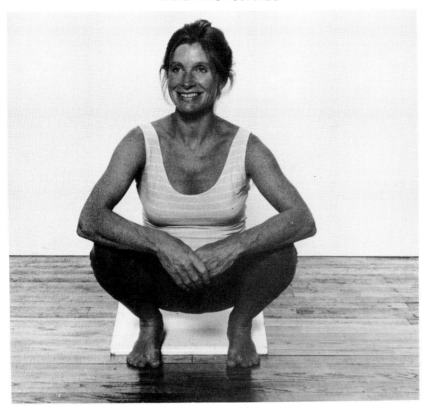

**4.14** Squatting

arms and trunk, as illustrated in Fig. 4.15. This stretch creates plenty of space in the uterus for the baby, and it is more stimulating for the abdomen than the same stretch done in Baddha Konasana (p. 45) or Virasana (p. 36). Sitting cross-legged is a good position in which to stretch the arms up and work on the shoulders, since it prevents one from hollowing the back excessively and from pushing the ribs too far forward.

The full Lotus pose is difficult for most Western people, so proceed gently and patiently, listen to your body and avoid forcing it.

To practise Padmasana, sit in an easy, cross-legged position, with a blanket or wedge under the buttocks if necessary to stop the pelvis from tilting back; your weight should be taken on the front of the buttock bones. With both hands take hold of your right foot and ankle and, keeping your right leg relaxed, lift the foot as high as possible, feeling the movement in the right hip joint. Turn the sole of the right foot towards you, moving the right knee forward and in towards the left knee. Then place the right foot on top of the left thigh close in to the groin, so that the right knee rests on the left foot. This is the Half Lotus posture. Make sure that the right foot is well supported on the left thigh, not sliding off so that only the toes rest on it.

Attempt the full Lotus pose only if the Half Lotus is comfortable, with the right

55

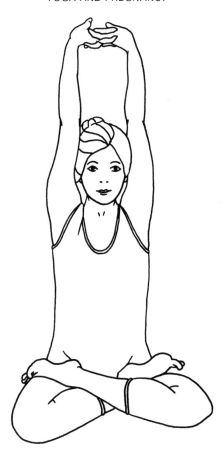

**4.15** Padmasana

knee easily touching the left foot. If the right knee is up in the air, or if the position is painful, then continue practising this position until it becomes comfortable, alternating the position of the legs.

To continue with Padmasana, lift up your left foot and place it, without forcing, on top of the right thigh, bringing the left knee in towards the right knee as far as possible. Extend the left knee away from the hip joint towards the floor. Make sure that you are sitting on the buttock bones (you can pull the flesh of the buttocks out of the way with your hands, as in the other sitting postures), and that your spine is stretching up evenly, without hollowing the back or sticking out the front ribs or chest. Keep your shoulders and arms relaxed, hands resting on your thighs, and extend the back of your neck, with your chin in.

Now interlock your fingers and stretch your arms out in front of you with outturned palms. Making a wide arc with your hands, take your arms above your head. Hold this position for a few breaths, then relax your arms, uncross your legs

56

and repeat the whole posture, reversing the position of the legs and the interlocked fingers.

### Crossed-knee Pose

This position is helpful as a preparation for Padmasana, and also as a way of preventing and relieving sciatic pain, which some women experience during pregnancy. Sit down with your left leg bent in front of you, the knee in line with your chest, the outer part of your left foot on the floor (see Fig. 4.16). Now cross

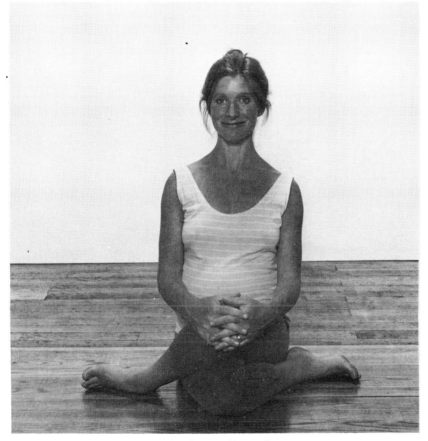

**4.16**   Crossed-knee Pose

the right leg over the left as far as it will go, so that the two knees are in line with each other and the right foot is as far back as the left. You may find this difficult at first, but you can practise it safely as long as you do not try to force the legs into position, and it will gradually become easier. Clasp the upper knee with your hands and make the feet alive, spreading the toes, to help you stretch the spine up well.

Repeat the pose with the position of the legs reversed.

## *Virasana, Hero Pose*

This posture is important because it forms a counter-pose to the other basic sitting and squatting poses, ensuring a balanced development of the legs and hips. The hip and knee joints are rotated inwards rather than outwards, counter-balancing the stretching that takes place in the cross-legged poses. Virasana is a good posture for improving flat feet (note how the tops of the feet are well stretched) and, together with the variation, Supta Virasana, helps to prevent and alleviate varicose veins. Both poses improve the circulation in the legs and are very restful after long periods of standing. They also help to relieve indigestion and heart-burn and are the only postures which can be practised with benefit immediately after a meal. Virasana is a useful sitting position for everyday use, and one which children adopt naturally when sitting on the floor.

To practise Virasana, start by kneeling up, with your knees together and your feet apart, the tops of your feet resting on the floor (see Fig. 4.17). Sit down gently between your feet, holding your ankles and taking your weight on your hands at first, if you are not sure whether you can sit on the floor without hurting your knees. If your knees or ankles are too stiff or painful for you to sit on the floor place

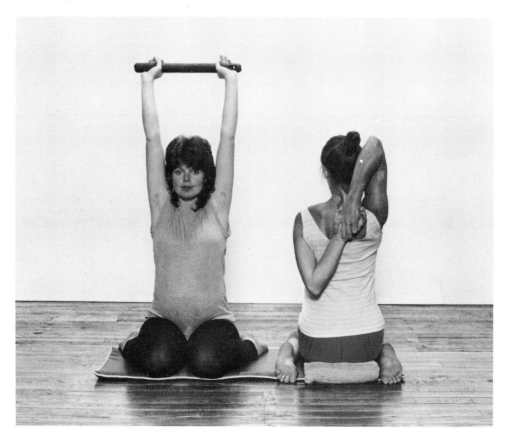

**4.17** Virasana

a folded blanket or a couple of telephone directories under your hips (see figure on the right). As you sit down, pull your calf muscles sideways out of the way of your thighs with your hands. Make sure that the tops of your feet rest on the ground. If your ankles hurt, do not turn your feet out sideways, but raise the height of the hips to take pressure off them. Make sure that your knees are level with each other and that you are sitting evenly on the two buttock bones. Keep your pelvis level and let your spine stretch up freely.

For a lovely stretch in the trunk, shoulders and arms, clasp a heavy stick (the one in the photograph is made of iron) and stretch it above your head. Alternatively, interlock your fingers and stretch your arms up, as illustrated in Padmasana, p. 56.

The position of the arms demonstrated by the woman on the right (Gomukasana) is an exercise for loosening the shoulders and the top part of the spine. You will find this position very valuable if you practise it regularly during pregnancy and after the birth. Carrying your baby and breast feeding can pull your shoulders forward and stiffen the upper back, if you do not give this area some careful attention. The advantage of this shoulder exercise is that it can be done at any time of day, whether you are standing, sitting or kneeling.

Stretch your right arm above your head, extending it well from shoulder to fingertips. Bend your right elbow and reach down your back with your right hand. At this point you can use your left hand to push the right elbow down a little. Now stretch your left arm out sideways at shoulder level, bend your left elbow and try to clasp your hands behind your back. Hold the position for a few moments, trying to bring your wrists closer to each other, then release your hands and repeat, reversing the position of the arms.

*Note*: if you cannot make your fingers meet behind your back, then clasp a piece of cloth about the size of a flannel with both your hands, gradually reducing the distance between them.

## Supta Virasana

This is a refreshing, restful posture which opens the chest and rib-cage and facilitates deep breathing. In early pregnancy, if you are very supple, you can lie back flat on the floor with your arms stretched behind your head, a position which puts a marvellous stretch on the front of the abdomen and the front thighs. However, in the later months it is better to place pillows or blankets under your back (see Fig. 4.18), in order to open the chest and to avoid straining the lower back or over-stretching the abdomen. If you have difficulty keeping your knees on the floor, you can rest them on a support, as shown.

To practise Supta Virasana, start in Virasana, with your blankets or cushions within reach. Hold your feet and lower yourself backwards until you are resting your weight on your elbows. At this point, tilt your pelvis in such a way that your coccyx moves away from your head towards your knees and your pubic bone moves nearer to your head. This movement is extremely important, otherwise there will be strain on your over-arched lumbar spine. If at this stage you find it

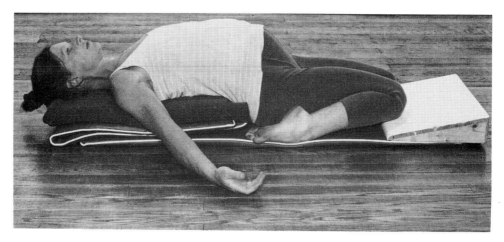

**4.18** Supta Virasana

difficult to keep your knees on the ground, pull a blanket or wedge underneath them. Now pull your other blankets or cushions behind your hips and slowly lie back on them. Relax your shoulders, arms, head and neck, and rest in this position with deep breathing for as long as is comfortable. You can stay in this pose for several minutes if you find it relaxing.

To come up, lift yourself on to your elbows first, then sit up on an inhalation.

### Ustrasana, Camel Pose

If you are already familiar with this posture, you can continue practising it for as long as you like, up to the end of pregnancy if it is comfortable. It gives a releasing stretch to the spine and the front of the body, as well as opening the chest and shoulder area. However, if you are a beginner, or if you find back bends a strain, then do not do this pose after the fourth month. Instead, you can practise Setu Bandha Sarvangasana (see p. 74) if you want to include a back bend in your yoga session.

To practise Ustrasana, kneel with your knees hip width apart and your feet the same distance apart, so that your lower legs are parallel. Have the tops of your feet resting on the floor (see Fig. 4.19). Stretch your spine up, keeping your coccyx tucked firmly down and in, so as to lengthen the lumbar. Bending back from your hips, place your hands against the backs of your thighs and slide them down towards the backs of the knees. You should feel that you are stretching your spine from as low as possible, rather than bending it in the middle; so to this end, keep your tail-bone tucked in (with the same movement of the pelvis as in Supta Virasana). If you can reach the backs of your knees easily, then reach back with one hand after the other to catch hold of your heels. Have your arms turned out

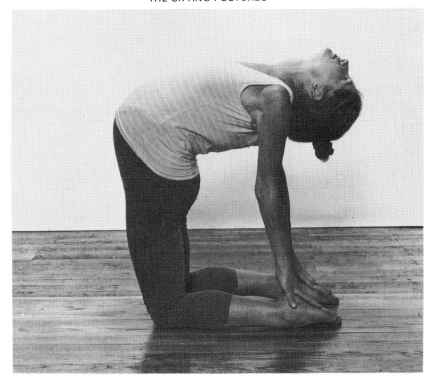

**4.19** Ustrasana

from the shoulders so that your thumbs are on the outside. Let your head drop
back gently so that your neck is stretched, and relax your breathing as you hold the
posture for not more than twenty seconds, lifting your breast-bone high towards
the ceiling.

Inhale as you come up slowly to the kneeling position, then rest on your heels.
To ease the back, follow Ustrasana with the kneeling forward bend (p. 53), the
squatting position (p. 55), or a twisting posture (see p. 62).

## Two Twisting Poses

The twisting postures keep the spine flexible and healthy, stimulating the many
nerves along the spinal column. They have a soothing effect and are often very
effective in relieving backache. In addition, they tone the abdominal muscles.

In the first four months of pregnancy you can practise any of the twisting
postures, but thereafter you have to avoid the ones that squash the abdomen. Both
the poses shown here can be done right to the end of pregnancy because they leave
the front of the body free and open. The first one puts a gentle twist on the
spine, the second is more intense.

### Bharadvajasana II

This posture (see Fig. 4.20, figure on left) puts a fairly gentle twist on the spine and

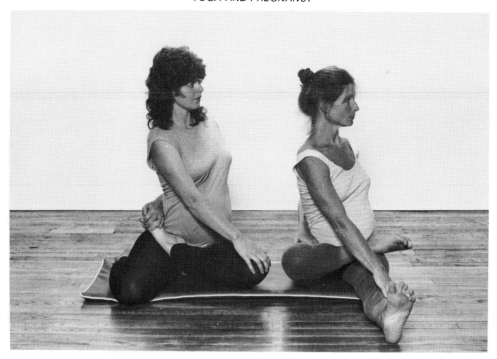

**4.20** Bharadvajasana II; Ardha Matsyendrasana II

is a lovely pose to do in late pregnancy because it feels balanced and stable, and, with the knees apart, the front of the body remains open and unconstricted. One leg is placed in Virasana, Hero Pose, the other in Padmasana, Lotus Pose. If you are unable to place the leg in Lotus, you can bend it to the side along with the other leg, so that you are sitting with both legs bent to one side.

Begin by sitting in Dandasana, then bend your right leg back as if for Virasana, the top of your right foot on the floor beside your right hip. Bring your left foot towards you, bending your left knee, and lift it up with your hands and place it on top of your right thigh, as for Padmasana. If you cannot do this, simply tuck your left ankle under your right thigh so that both legs are folded to the right. Place your right hand on your left knee, keeping your right arm straight, and sit tall, extending your spine out of the pelvis. Exhaling, twist slowly to the left, keeping your shoulders down, your chest open and your back stretching up all the time. Walk the fingertips of your left hand around behind you, and then catch the toes of your left foot with that hand.

Hold the twist for a few moments with normal breathing, then release your foot and stretch your legs out before repeating it to the other side, reversing the position of the legs.

*Ardha Matsyendrasana II*
This is a useful pose if you wish to put a stronger twist on the spine (see Fig. 4.20,

figure on right). It is suitable only if you can place your legs comfortably in Padmasana, and if your spine is very flexible; therefore it is not for beginners.

Start in Dandasana, then bend your right knee and place your right leg in the Lotus position, as described for Padmasana (see p. 56). Keep your left leg stretched out, spreading your toes and extending the left heel firmly away from you. Sit with a straight back, with your weight well forward on the buttock bones. With an exhalation, twist round to the left until you can catch hold of your right thigh with your left hand. Rest your right hand on your outstretched left leg and use it to help you turn your trunk further to the left. Do not tense your shoulders; lift your breast-bone and keep your chest broad and open.

Hold this position with normal breathing, then release the thigh and stretch out your right leg before repeating the pose to the other side.

## Chapter 5

# The Inverted Postures and Pelvic-floor Exercises

## The inverted postures

The postures in this section should not be attempted if you are a beginner in yoga, with the possible exception of Sarvangasana, Shoulderstand, if you are starting early in pregnancy. If you are accustomed to practising the inverted postures, then you can continue doing them through most or all of your pregnancy, with great benefit to you and your baby. It is worth emphasising again that there are no fixed rules as to when various postures should be discontinued, since it varies from one individual to another. The only 'rule' is that your body should be well balanced, well aligned, with plenty of space created for the internal organs and the baby. The word 'asana', meaning seat, implies that the posture should be stable and promote a sense of ease. Some women will find that this is true of Headstand, for example, until the day of the birth, whereas others will want to discontinue it at six or seven months. It is important to be guided by your own body, for it all depends *how* you do the pose.

The benefits of the inverted postures are the same during pregnancy as at other times – the reversed pull of gravity improves circulation and regulates the functioning of the glands and the internal organs. Because of the way in which they affect the glands and hormone production, the inverted postures can help to protect against miscarriage. They minimise the chances of suffering from many of the problems commonly associated with pregnancy, such as varicose veins, constipation and insomnia. They counteract any heavy, downward dragging feeling from the weight of the baby pressing on the pelvic floor. And when you do these postures, it often feels as though they have a stimulating effect on the baby itself.

### Adho Mukha Vrksasana, Full Arm Balance

The Sanskrit name of this posture means Upside Down Tree Pose, and it gives a similar stretch through the entire body, with the added benefits of inversion. The arms and shoulders are strengthened, the neck completely relaxed, circulation is improved, and the weight of the baby is taken off the pelvis and legs. It is a fairly strenuous posture to hold for long, so in the later months maintain it for only a few seconds at a time.

To practise Adho Mukha Vrksasana, bend one knee so that you can place your hands on the floor, two or three inches away from the wall. Your hands should be the same width apart as your shoulders, and your other leg should be straight, with the foot further back than that of the bent leg, rather as if you were preparing to sprint. Keeping your arms straight, swing your straight leg firmly up to the wall, letting your other leg follow (see Fig. 5.1). Do not bend your elbows or let your shoulders collapse. Let your neck and head hang loosely and breathe normally. Keep distance between your ears and shoulders by moving your shoulders away

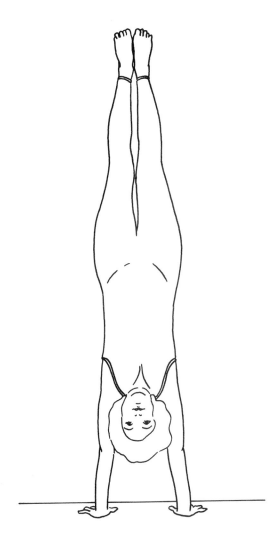

**5.1**  Adho Mukha Vrksasana

from the floor, keep your tail-bone tucked in so that you do not hollow your back, and stretch up the wall as if trying to lift your heels nearer to the ceiling.

To come down, bend one leg and lower it gently to the ground, letting your other leg follow. Keep all your movements as smooth and controlled as possible. After completing the posture, do not stand up too quickly.

## *Salamba Sirsasana, Headstand*

When it is well executed, this posture feels marvellous throughout pregnancy. Headstand is an active, exhilarating pose which brings mental clarity and a positive frame of mind. Together with Shoulderstand, it can be of great value in the early months of pregnancy when there may be feelings of nausea and lethargy. A good Headstand is held more by balance than muscular effort, and the body adjusts gradually to the increase in weight as the baby grows, so you can expect to be able to practise it without difficulty for the full nine months. It is essential to have practised Headstand for some time before becoming pregnant, so that you have learned to maintain the necessary lift in the shoulders; otherwise, the extra weight of the baby could place strain on the neck; there is no strain on the neck when the posture is done correctly. Figure 5.2 shows how the pole can be used to check your alignment, in the same way as for Tadasana. This is important, since if you are out of alignment, there will be strain on your back, just as there is if you stand on your feet with poor posture. If you have no one to help you, practise Headstand sometimes by an outer corner where two walls meet. Instead of clasping your hands, place the palms of your hands against the walls near the corner, so that you are 'holding' the corner, and use the vertical edge to straighten the back of your body against. Failing that, use an inner corner, keeping your hands clasped in the usual Headstand position.

To practise Sirsasana, fold your blanket to form a smooth even pad large enough to accommodate your head and forearms. If you are practising without assistance in the second half of pregnancy, it is wise to practise by a wall in case of falling. Kneel on all fours and place your forearms on your blanket with your elbows shoulder width apart and level with each other, and with your fingers interlocked. Now let your head hang loosely from your neck above the place where you will rest the crown of your head. Having relaxed and lengthened your neck, gently lower your head to the blanket. Now straighten your legs and, resting lightly on your toes, walk your feet towards your head until your hips are directly in line with your shoulders, back straight. Lift your shoulders firmly away from the floor and let your spine stretch up. Now, without jumping, gently bend your knees so that your feet leave the floor, and draw them up, bringing your heels near your buttocks, being careful not to disturb your balance. Finally straighten your legs, and check that you have not collapsed your shoulders (see Fig. 5.2).

Lift your whole body by feeling your head, wrists and elbows pressing against the ground and pushing up from there. Stretch upwards through your shoulders, spine, legs and feet. Spread your toes and stretch the inner legs well. Be careful not

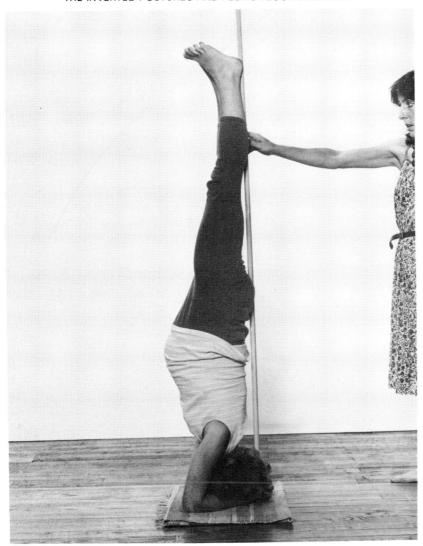

**5.2** Sirsasana

to let your tail-bone stick out, so that the small of your back hollows. Try to stand in Headstand as you do in Tadasana. Relax your fingers; relax your face and throat – you should be able to talk easily in this position. Stretch your legs up actively to help lift the weight of the pelvis off the lumbar spine; the more you stretch up, the lighter the pose becomes.

Stay in Headstand for as long as your balance feels good. If you begin to need much muscular effort to hold it, then it is time to come down. Bend your knees and lower your legs to the half-way position, then unfold your legs and lower them gently to the ground. Rest your knees on the floor and stay for a few moments in a kneeling position, keeping your head on the floor and relaxing your neck and shoulders. Then stretch your arms out in front of you along the floor and move your knees further apart, so that you are in the kneeling forward-bend. Finally, inhale as you sit up.

After completing Headstand, you may like to do Svanasana, Dog Pose, which stretches the spine and relaxes the neck while keeping the shoulders open (see p. 16).

If you practise Headstand, always practise Shoulderstand as well. Headstand should precede Shoulderstand and should not be practised without it. However, Shoulderstand can be practised without Headstand, and indeed should be mastered before Headstand is attempted.

## *Two variations of Sirsasana*

These two variations of Sirsasana are pleasant to do during pregnancy. In the first, spread your legs wide apart, as for Upavistha Konasana (see Fig. 5.3); in the second, place your legs in Baddha Konasana (see Fig. 5.4). Try to move your legs without disturbing your upper body: do not let your elbows slide out or your shoulders collapse; make sure that you do not collapse the lumbar spine or turn the hips; and keep your tail-bone tucked in. In Baddha Konasana, move your knees as far back as possible to open the hips.

Straighten your legs and bring them together before coming down.

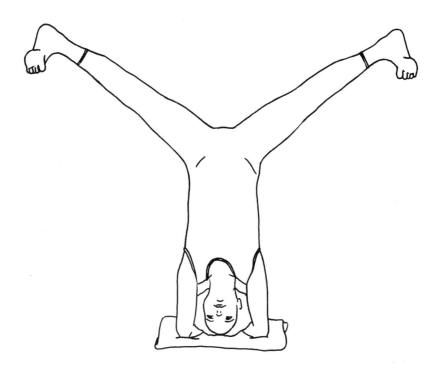

**5.3**  Sirsasana, variation

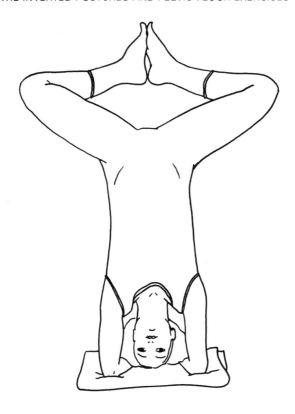

**5.4** Sirsasana, variation

## Salamba Sarvangasana, Shoulderstand or Neck Balance

Like Headstand, Shoulderstand can be practised until the end of pregnancy, with great benefit to the spine, the circulation, the internal organs, and to your mental state. It is a quiet, calming, inward-looking posture, complementing Headstand, which is more stimulating and outward-looking. Shoulderstand requires more muscular effort to hold a good vertical position, and you are more likely to feel your increasing weight as a hindrance in this pose. If you find that you cannot hold it without strain, then try using a chair for support (see p. 73). Less experienced students may find that they have to discontinue practice of Shoulderstand altogether before the end of the pregnancy, though Halasana with the legs supported may still be comfortable. Continue practising these asanas only as long as your body is in balance and they leave you feeling well and refreshed.

Figure 5.6 shows Sarvangasana done in the ninth month of pregnancy. However, depending on your weight and build, as well as the amount of yoga experience you have, you may wish to practise with the support of a chair at any time after about five months. For the first four months at least, you can practise the pose without support. Have your blanket folded evenly, as for Headstand, with

69

another blanket or two underneath, similarly folded, to give extra height under your shoulders. This is important, since your neck should be as relaxed as possible, with space beneath it; it should not be pressed into the floor. Your folded blanket must be large enough to accommodate your shoulders, upper arms and elbows easily.

*Halasana, Plough Pose* (part of the Shoulderstand sequence)
Lie down in such a way that your shoulders are in line with the edge of your blankets, and the back of your head is on the floor, keeping a gap between the back of your neck and the ground. Have a chair behind your head, two or three feet away. With an exhalation, raise your legs, either keeping them straight, or (later in pregnancy) bending your knees; then, pressing your arms into the floor by your sides, lift your hips and roll over, bringing your legs behind your head and lifting your back right off the floor. Straighten your legs and rest your feet on the chair behind you (see Fig. 5.5). In the early months you can rest your feet on the floor or on a low stool or pile of books, providing that you can keep your back straight. However supple you are, you will have to rest your feet on a chair after a few months to avoid squashing the uterus. There must be enough space between your thighs and your chest to allow the baby plenty of room.

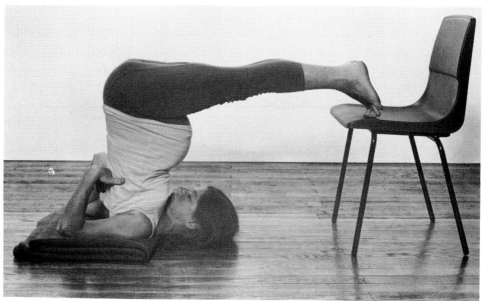

**5.5** Halasana

While in Halasana, try to lift yourself right on to the tops of the shoulders, so that your shoulder blades are off the floor. To help this, interlock your fingers behind your back and, exhaling, stretch your arms out along the floor with your palms facing your back. At the end of this movement, lift your whole spine from the ground. Without letting your elbows slide out wider than your shoulders, place your hands on your back and support it just above the shoulder blades with your

70

thumbs and forefingers. Increase the stretch in your spine by lifting your buttock bones upwards. Stretch the backs of the legs thoroughly by extending your heels away from your hips and lifting the backs of your knees and thighs towards the ceiling. Your knees should be quite straight, while your hips should be directly above your shoulders, so that your spine is vertical. Your feet should be resting very lightly on the tips of your toes on the chair. Breathe normally, allowing the spine and the backs of the legs to lengthen on every exhalation.

To come up into Sarvangasana, support your back firmly with your hands to prevent your chest moving away from your chin, and raise your legs to the vertical position with an exhalation. You can either keep your legs straight throughout, or bend your knees and then straighten them again. In Shoulderstand, your legs should be vertical, with your feet and ankles above your shoulders (see Fig. 5.6). If your legs lean over your head, this may put strain on your neck, especially in pregnancy when you are heavier than usual. If in doubt, ask a friend to tell you if you are straight, or to check your position using the pole, as in Headstand (see Fig. 5.2).

Stay in Sarvangasana, breathing normally, for as long as is comfortable. Stretch your legs and feet up, as if trying to stand upon the ceiling. Keep your face and throat relaxed and let your tongue relax, so that it is not pressing against the roof of your mouth.

From Shoulderstand, return to Halasana by lowering your feet to the chair on an exhalation, supporting your back firmly so that your spine does not collapse. From Halasana, roll your spine down to the floor, letting your legs follow. To control the descent, stretch your arms out along the floor behind your back, palms down, and walk your hands away from you as you come down. After completing Halasana and Sarvangasana, practise Setu Bandha Sarvangasana (p. 73).

*Sarvangasana with the support of a chair*
When you begin to feel that you need some support in Shoulderstand, try it with a chair propping your hips, as shown in Fig. 5.7. It is somewhat complicated to get into position on your own, but it is worth the trouble because you are then able to hold the posture with ease for longer than usual. You need two chairs, one behind your head to rest your feet on in Halasana, and one near your hips that you can pull towards you when you are ready to lift up into Shoulderstand.

First of all, move into Halasana, resting your toes on the seat of the chair. When in Halasana, reach out for your other chair and draw it close to your hips with the front edge of the seat touching your back. Stretching your arms behind your back, thread them through the *inside* of the front legs to hold the back legs of the chair. With an exhalation, raise your legs until they are vertical, resting your hips against the seat of the chair, as shown. You will feel more stable if you work with the chair against a wall so that it cannot slide away. If you have a friend to help you, she can move the chairs into position for you as you need them.

To come down, lower your feet to the chair behind your head, returning to Halasana, push the chair behind your back out of the way, and roll your spine

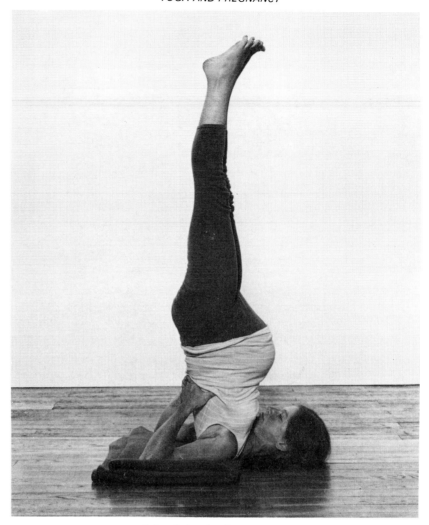

**5.6** Salamba Sarvangasana

gently down to the floor, making sure the palms of your hands are flat on the ground behind you.

*Note*: a very restful version of Halasana can be done with your legs completely supported on a chair or piece of furniture of similar height. Have the lower part of your legs, from feet to knees, resting on the support, with a cushion under your legs for greater comfort. If your chair has a solid back like the one shown here, you will have to turn it sideways. After stretching your back up well, you can extend your arms behind your head along the floor, towards your feet. Use this as a relaxing position; it should be comfortable to hold for five or ten minutes even at the end of pregnancy.

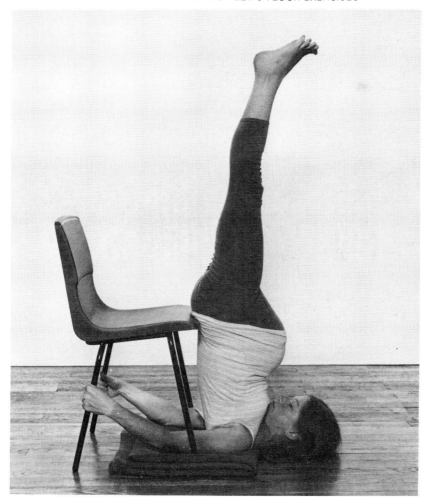

**5.7** Salamba Sarvangasana, supported

## *Setu Bandha Sarvangasana, Bridging Pose*

Do this pose immediately after Sarvangasana. It relaxes your neck, opens your chest and rib-cage beautifully, and provides a gentle back-bend to counter-balance the forward-bending position of Halasana. Normally this posture is done as part of the Shoulderstand sequence by dropping the feet to the ground from Sarvangasana. However, this is not recommended after the first four months of pregnancy, and it can be done instead by lifting the hips and back up from the floor.

After rolling down from Sarvangasana, bend your knees up, drawing your feet towards your hips. Keep your feet flat on the floor, parallel and hip width apart (see Fig. 5.8). On no account let your feet turn out; there is often a strong tendency for this to happen, so, if in doubt, turn the toes slightly inwards. Press your big toe joints into the floor and lift the inner edges of the feet. With an exhalation, lift your

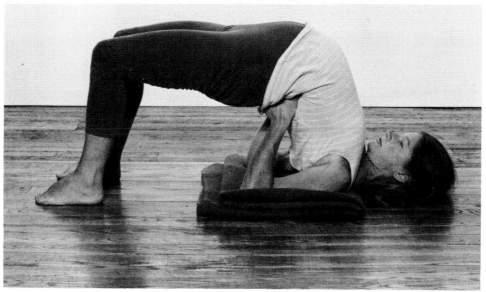

**5.8** Setu Bandha Sarvangasana

hips from the floor, keeping your tail-bone tucked in, but without squeezing your buttock muscles tightly together. Raise your pelvis as high as you can, supporting your back with your hands in the same way as for Sarvangasana. Move your elbows further in towards each other, lift your ribs and shoulder blades up from the floor and keep your heels firmly on the ground.

Breathing normally, hold this position for as long as is comfortable, then lower your spine gently to the floor as shown in Fig. 5.9, trying to place one vertebra down at a time. Relax, with your knees still bent and your lower spine flat on the

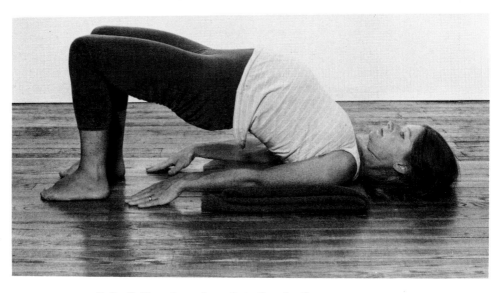

**5.9** Rolling down from Setu Bandha Sarvangasana

floor, before straightening your legs. Keep your knees bent up if your lower back aches, and wait until the ache disappears before stretching your legs out. Roll on to your side before sitting up.

## Pelvic-floor Exercises

The condition of the pelvic-floor muscles is crucial for a woman's health at all times, though she may only become aware of them at or after the birth of her first child. The pelvic floor acts as a support for the internal organs, and a weak pelvic floor can lead to many disorders, from incontinence to prolapse of the uterus. Like the abdominal muscles, with which they are closely linked, the pelvic-floor muscles can become badly weakened and overstretched from the additional strain of pregnancy and birth, unless they are adequately exercised. Weak pelvic-floor muscles increase the likelihood of needing an episiotomy at birth – that is, a cut made in the perineum to enlarge the opening and ease delivery. Episiotomies are performed with alarming frequency, often unnecessarily, with long-term after-effects of discomfort or pain, so it is worth making sure that your muscles are in good shape and that you present your midwife or doctor with every reason not to perform this rather brutal operation.

Strong muscles are not necessarily tight muscles. A strong, healthy muscle, well supplied with blood and oxygen from frequent exercise, has the ability to stretch without strain or tearing, and to spring back afterwards to its previous shape, like elastic. When exercising the muscles of the pelvic floor, you practise contracting and releasing them, increasing both their strength and their suppleness. As a preparation for birth, learning to let go of these muscles is as important as being able to contract them, for it is essential to relax them during the second stage of labour, when the baby's head emerges.

Many women have so little awareness of this part of their bodies that they have no control of the muscles at all at first. But regular practise brings awareness and control quite quickly, for, fortunately, these muscles respond promptly to exercise, and it is never too late to improve their condition. Simply being aware of the pelvic-floor muscles means that you will be able to release them consciously at the moment of birth. A rigid pelvic floor, which can impede the birth and result in injury, is usually due to tension arising from fear and ignorance. Most women experience fear or apprehension at some point during labour, but the more bodily awareness you have, the more easily you will recognise defensive tightening up in certain areas of the body, including the perineum, and be able to relax them deliberately.

Pelvic-floor exercises are so simple that they can easily be incorporated into both your yoga practice and your daily life, without having to set aside a special time for them. Once you are familiar with the exercises, make it a habit to practise them at odd moments during the day – when you are brushing your teeth, queueing in shops or waiting at traffic lights in the car. Since they should be done little and often every day, this is a sensible way of approaching them.

During your yoga practice, you can make a point of drawing up the pelvic-floor muscles while in Sarvangasana, Shoulderstand. This is easier if you place the heel of one foot on top of the toes of the other foot, so that your legs are slightly crossed. Alternate the position of the legs, and repeat. Discover how different postures affect the pelvic floor. For instance, in the squatting position, which should be practised often during pregnancy, it is easy to release the pelvic-floor muscles. In Virasana, or when kneeling, it is easy to contract them, drawing them up into the body.

To familiarise yourself with the pelvic-floor muscles, start practising the basic exercise in a comfortable lying position – the bath is an ideal place. If the muscles are weak, it is better to start exercising them while lying down, so that you are not working against gravity. Place one hand on the pubic bone and draw up the pelvic-floor muscles, so as to tighten all the internal passages. Imagine your vagina tightening as high as the level of your hand. Hold for a few seconds, then relax. Do this up to five times in succession, as often as you can. Make sure that you do.not tense the muscles of the abdomen, buttocks or thighs instead of the pelvic floor, and that you do not hold your breath while contracting the muscles; keep your breathing relaxed.

A very effective variation of this exercise is to contract and release the muscles in stages, holding at each level for a second or two, and aiming to include four levels of contraction. The analogy of a lift stopping at four floors on its way up and down is useful. Being able to pause on the way down is a real test of control of the pelvic floor.

A useful way of incorporating pelvic-floor exercises into everyday life is to practise stopping the flow of urine every time you go to the lavatory, except perhaps first thing in the morning if this is a strain. And become aware of the pelvic floor at other times, especially after any bearing down movement, such as a bowel movement, coughing, sneezing, laughing, or lifting a heavy object. Always follow such a movement with a strong uplifting pelvic floor contraction.

*Chapter 6*

# Relaxation and Breathing

'During pregnancy yoga helped strengthen my back and also helped me to relax. I wanted to carry on with yoga when pregnant, because I thought it important to keep my body supple. I had a long and difficult delivery, but I felt I was able to handle it by practising the relaxing I'd learnt from Yoga.'

*Fran*

'The most important posture of all, and the one that helped me most to be able to relax during the birth, was Savasana [Corpse Pose]. The actual birth was so easy – he just seemed to fall out, I'm sure that was because I'd opened up a lot doing yoga.'

*Amanda*

'Having done breath control in yoga for two years any birth class breathing was a cinch. Relaxing and breathing through early contractions is helpful.'

*Tessa*

One of the greatest benefits of yoga during pregnancy is learning to relax consciously and deliberately. The increased bodily awareness that yoga brings enables you to notice unnecessary tension arising in any situation. Certain parts of the body, such as the neck, shoulders and jaw, seem to be especially prone to tension. If you observe yourself carefully while you are engaged in any activity, you will soon discover which are your particular tension spots. A great deal of energy can be wasted through this kind of unnecessary muscular tension, which, when it is habitual, can lead to permanent distortion of posture, fatigue and pain. Through yoga we learn to dissociate different parts of the body, so that those not directly involved in any particular activity can be relaxed. This ability releases energy for the task in hand.

Relaxation is an invaluable skill for coping with all kinds of stress, and various forms of stress are encountered during the child-bearing year. Pregnancy makes extra demands on the body and can make a woman emotionally more vulnerable than usual; the stress of birth is brief and intense; after the birth there is the continuing day-to-day stress of caring for a young baby in addition to your normal work, and coping with the sudden changes in your body, as well as sheer fatigue from the whole birth experience and sleep deprivation afterwards. The ability to relax is essential for a straightforward, natural birth, since tension, from physical or emotional causes, can disrupt the birth process. Should some unforeseen complication arise during labour, if you are able to relax and to trust in your body's powers of recovery, you improve your chances of a safe and positive experience, with or without the help of medical intervention.

Every yoga session should end with five or ten minutes (or longer) in Savasana, Corpse Pose, the posture of complete relaxation of the body, mind and breath. Ideally, Savasana should be done every day, even on those days when you miss the rest of your yoga practice, but it is easier to do when you have worked at the other asanas first, so that your muscles are already well stretched and slightly fatigued. Pregnancy is a very good time to cultivate the habit of daily relaxation. It is a time when you are encouraged to take plenty of rest, and it is a time when you probably feel naturally disposed to sitting or lying down quietly and turning your attention inwards. The growing baby can help to develop a sense of centre which may be elusive at other times; the feeling of increasing weight and life in the pelvis and lower abdomen makes you very conscious of this area of the body.

A sense of strength and firmness in the physical centre is associated, in yoga and other eastern disciplines, with psychological stability. If you are a person who normally finds it difficult to sit or lie quietly doing nothing, because your brain is too busy, you may find it easier during pregnancy to drop your consciousness away from your head to the centre of your body. With this can come a feeling of peace and stillness, of an enduring centre, and even a complete change of perspective on life. One of the joys of pregnancy is to experience life shaping itself in and through yourself, something over which you have no conscious control and to which you have to surrender completely. It is this surrender to life that yoga relaxation helps to bring about, but which can be difficult for people who live in their heads, alienated from their instincts, and who may be afraid of letting go of what they believe is their control over events. If you do find it hard to take time off for relaxation, you can start by reminding yourself that lying down in Savasana is benefiting not only yourself, but your baby too.

## Savasana, Corpse Pose

Practise Savasana at the end of your yoga practice, preferably after a soothing posture such as a forward-bend, Sarvangasana, Halasana, or perhaps a twisting pose. Spread your blanket out on the floor so that when you lie down your whole body can be on it. Sit down first, then lie on your back with your knees bent up and your feet flat on the floor (see Fig. 6.1, figure at the back). If your back aches, bend your knees towards your chest (keeping your knees apart in the later months) and hug them against you, or even rock gently backwards and forwards on your spine. Then place your feet flat on the floor again, hip width apart and parallel, your knees in the air. If your neck and shoulders are tight, place a book under the back of your head. For the brain to become quiet, your throat must be relaxed, with your chin level, not jutting in the air; the book helps to achieve this.

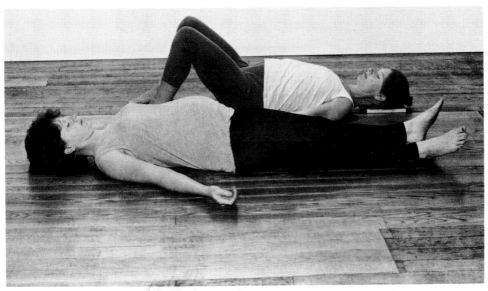

**6.1** Savasana

The back of your neck should be elongated, bringing your chin in. Try picking up your head with both hands and gently stretching your neck, then place your head back on the floor, keeping it straight, so that it rests as near to the base of the skull as possible. It is even better if you can get someone else to do this for you. Now stretch your arms out from your shoulders and rest them on the floor with the palms of your hands facing upwards. Lift your shoulder blades very slightly from the floor and shift them towards your feet, so that the front edge of each shoulder moves a little nearer to the ground (this is the same action as that of the shoulders in all the other asanas, when they are dropped down and back, away from the ears). As you do this, your top chest lifts a little. Your lower ribs should not lift up, but should relax down and sideways as you breathe. Move your tail-bone towards your feet to flatten your lumbar spine against the floor. Keep your feet flat, turning neither in nor out, with your knees directly above your feet. Stay in this position until your lumbar spine feels completely relaxed – just let it release into the floor. At the same time, let go of your head, neck, shoulders, arms, rib-cage and upper back. When you feel that all tension has disappeared from the small of your back, carefully stretch your legs out one after the other, keeping your tail-bone moving towards your feet and the pelvis broad and relaxed. If your lower back immediately arches up off the floor, you should continue your relaxation with your knees bent up, or, better still, with your lower legs resting on a chair or a bed.

Close your eyes and let your eyeballs become relaxed and heavy, sinking back into your head. Feel the back of your body in contact with the ground. Seek out areas of tension and release them. Think of the ground moving up underneath you, supporting you completely. Give yourself up totally to gravity, to the earth, and keep your awareness in the back of your body. You should feel yourself broadening and lengthening as your softening skin lets go, rather like a spilled liquid spreading out on the floor. Let the skin of your face smooth out from the centre to the sides, widening the space between the eyebrows, broadening the forehead, and softening the cheeks and the corners of the mouth. Experience a feeling of lightness between the brows. Let your hands, wrists, feet and ankles relax. Feel your bones becoming heavy and relaxed. Relax your brain.

Observe the way you are breathing. The more deeply you relax, the lighter and finer the breath becomes, with the exhalation longer than the inhalation. Do not try to control the breath; simply watch it going and coming of its own accord, as if something is breathing through you, through your pelvis and lower abdomen, the only noticeable movement being in the centre of the body, around the navel.

Stay very attentive, so that you notice when the mind wanders away from the body and the breath. Observe the thoughts as they arise, without judgement, and let them go, always taking your attention back to the breath. If you find this difficult, remind yourself of the contact between the back of your body and the ground, really experiencing it physically, then the brain will become quiet again. Make sure that your eyes are heavy and still and that your tongue is relaxed, so that it does not press against the roof of your mouth.

When you feel ready to come out of your deeply relaxed state, open your eyes without focusing them immediately. Look out as if from the back of your head. Stay lying quietly on the floor for a few moments, continuing to observe yourself and remaining aware of the back of your body. Notice how you feel. Notice how, by giving yourself up entirely to the earth, you have received energy from it and are restored. In the same way, the front of your body, which has been completely exposed and vulnerable, has been open to receive energy from the air. After a few moments, take a few deeper breaths and roll over on to your side. Stay like this for a few moments more before getting up. You may feel that this is an ideal time to just sit quietly, with your back completely straight, for five or ten minutes, before returning to your usual activities.

Comfort is essential in this pose, otherwise you will not be able to relax completely. Some women find that in later pregnancy they are uncomfortable lying flat on their back. The weight of the uterus pressing on major blood vessels and on the diaphragm can cause faintness. If you experience this, try placing cushions or folded blankets under your back as in Supta Virasana (see p. 59). If even this position is uncomfortable, you may prefer to lie on your side with your upper leg bent. Place a cushion under the bent knee, a small pillow under your head, and, if preferred, a cushion under the uterus. Bend one arm behind you and let it relax on the floor. Some women, on the other hand, experience no discomfort in the classic Corpse Pose, in which case it can be practised until the very end of pregnancy. The more yoga you have practised previously, the less likely you are to have problems with Savasana.

Always make sure that you are comfortably warm. Lie with your whole body on a blanket or carpet, and put on socks and an extra jersey after practising the asanas, unless it is a very warm day. It is surprising how quickly you can cool down when lying still, even if you feel warm to start with, and the floor is often a draughty place. Your clothes should be completely unrestricting, so if you put on extra clothes for warmth, leave them undone. Remove glasses or contact lenses before lying down.

## Deep breathing

Good, efficient deep breathing is extremely important for your own health and that of your baby during pregnancy. The way we breathe determines to a large extent our general health and sense of well-being. When we breathe fully, using the lower ribs and diaphragm as well as the upper chest, both the circulation of oxygen throughout the body and the removal of waste products are more thorough, improving many of the bodily functions. The action of the diaphragm in deep breathing also improves blood circulation, because the main vein from the lower body passes through it, and it has a very beneficial massaging action on the internal organs. The breathlessness that many women experience in later pregnancy can be avoided altogether by practising deep breathing exercises.

Deep breathing improves the condition of the heart and lungs, so that they function well during labour. If the diaphragm is properly exercised, it may help to speed up the second stage of labour, since the diaphragm assists the expulsive contractions of the uterus. And simply becoming aware of the breath helps you to release unnecessary tension during labour and to meet the sensations of the birth process and ride them instead of tightening up against them. Breathing thus helps you to open yourself to the experience of birth and to cope in a positive way with pain.

The keys to good breathing are posture and exercise. When we exercise vigorously, this automatically stimulates deep breathing – we are compelled to take in more oxygen and use our lungs to full capacity. Hence the value of continuing fairly strong exercise throughout pregnancy. However, there are many women who take almost no strenuous exercise on a regular basis, even when they are not pregnant, and whose breathing is probably shallow and inadequate. In such a case it is especially important to make time for some regular practice of deep breathing, in order to increase your awareness of the breath generally and to re-educate the chief muscles used in breathing, the diaphragm and the intercostal muscles. These muscles must have room to move. When posture is bad, with rounded, hunched shoulders and collapsed chest, space in the rib-cage is seriously constricted and deep breathing impossible. The asanas restore good posture by opening the chest, loosening stiff shoulders, and stretching and correcting distortion in the spine.

The breath is not only a vital ingredient of your physical health, but it forms a link between your body and your mind. If you are emotionally agitated, your breathing is affected. When you deliberately steady and relax your breathing, your mind becomes calm. And relaxing the body automatically relaxes the breath. So it becomes clear why both physical training (asanas) and breath control are closely linked with the practice of meditation. According to the classical yoga theory of

Patanjali, asana (posture) and pranayama (breath control) are prerequisites for the practice of concentration and contemplation.

*Posture for deep breathing*

A slumped spine leads to shallow breathing and a dull mind. The essential requirement for breathing exercises and meditation is that the spine should be erect and balanced, the shoulders directly above the hips. Any position that achieves this can be used. The classic position is the Lotus posture (Padmasana), because of its stability and symmetry. However, few Western people are able to sit comfortably in Padmasana for more than two or three minutes. For fairly supple people, the Half Lotus, in which one leg is folded on top of the other, is an excellent alternative (see p. 55). Figure 6.2 shows two simple ways of sitting that can be held

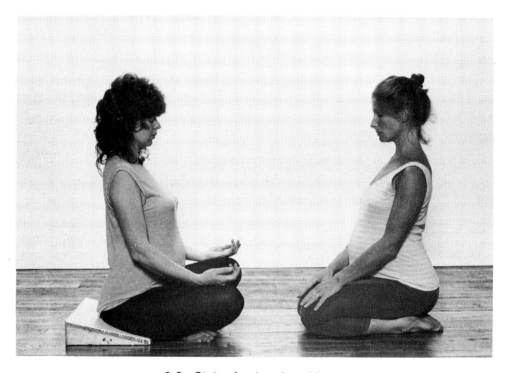

**6.2** Sitting for deep breathing

comfortably by most people for a few minutes. The simple cross-legged pose uses the wedge underneath the buttocks to lift the spine; this minimises strain in the back from holding the posture for any length of time. When sitting cross-legged, make sure to alternate the position of your legs regularly.

Having established the base of your posture – legs and pelvis – your spine should be able to stretch up in a perfectly balanced way, so that there is no sense of effort in the back muscles. This is possible when the body weight is taken on the buttock bones and when the shoulders are relaxed. Be aware of the bones rather than the muscles; imagine the spinal column, with the vertebrae balanced one above the other, resembling the stem of a plant growing upwards. Feel the top of your chest lifting and feel your shoulders dropping as you release tension in them. Let your arms relax, with your hands resting loosely on your knees, as shown. Alternatively, place your hands in your lap, palms up, one hand on top of the other. The weight of your arms should pull your shoulders down, but not cause your back to slump. Extend your neck upwards, with your chin in and the crown of your head uppermost.

Whenever you practise deep breathing, spend a few moments first finely adjusting your posture, and then observing your natural rhythm of breathing. For at least a minute keep your mind on your breath without controlling it, and notice what happens in your body as you breathe. As you inhale, a certain amount of tension enters the body, even when the breathing is light and relaxed, and when you exhale there is a tendency to drop the chest and sag slightly. When you breathe deeply, these tendencies become much more exaggerated, so you have to remain constantly aware of your posture as well as concentrating on the breath. As you inhale, do not let your shoulders lift or become tense; there is no need for them to move, since the rib-cage works independently of them. As you exhale, do not allow your top chest to collapse or your shoulders to come forward. You must maintain your erect posture throughout, but without unnecessary tension, and this takes a great deal of awareness and concentration. There is a kind of happy balance between going with the flow of the breath and keeping a firm and stable posture, the familiar combination in yoga of softness and firmness. These are Patanjali's words on posture: 'Asana [posture] implies steadiness and comfort. It requires relaxation and meditation on the Immovable. Then opposing sensations cease to torment.'

When you feel that you have reached a harmonious posture and state of mind, proceed with steady, deep breathing. Start by exhaling. Without collapsing your chest or spine, exhale smoothly and deeply, really emptying the lungs, feeling your rib-cage and abdomen contracting. Breathe out through your nose, keeping your nostrils and tongue relaxed and listening to the sound of the breath as it also passes through the mouth against the top palate. When you cannot exhale any more, but before the point of feeling strain, start letting the breath flow smoothly in again without a break. This time feel the air passing through the nose and mouth with a slightly different sound from that of the exhalation; feel your rib-cage expanding to the back, sides and front; feel your lungs filling with air, and check whether you are tensing your shoulders. Inhale smoothly and deliberately as deeply as you can without strain, then, without a break, start again on the exhalation.

Use the sound of the breath to ascertain whether you are breathing smoothly and rhythmically, and to time the length of the breaths. The inhalation and the exhalation should be of the same length. Most people find that their breath is irregular at first; in other words, they may find it easier to inhale deeply than to exhale deeply, or the other way around. Adjust the rate of breathing to match the shorter of the two, so that you are always working within your capacity. With practice, you will gradually extend your capacity, and you will also train yourself to become more balanced. Carry on with continuous deep breathing for as long as is comfortable. Your mind may wander, in which case simply become aware of it, and bring your attention back to the breath. If there is any physical strain or discomfort, you should stop and relax. This is important, as the breath is a very subtle thing. You should always feel good after deep breathing, then you will want to return to it. Forcing the breath can only be damaging. The feeling of well-being after good practice of deep breathing is unique: one feels totally refreshed and invigorated, very calm but very alive.

### Variations on the breath

When you are able to practise normal deep breathing with ease and enjoyment for several minutes, you can try these two variations which both involve retention of the breath. Normally this retention is done alternately on the in and the out breath, but in pregnancy it is not advisable to deprive oneself or the baby of oxygen even for a few seconds, so only the inhalation is held. Holding the breath in (without strain) is very beneficial as it ensures good circulation of oxygen to all parts of the body, including the baby.

1   After practising normal deep breathing for a few minutes, alter the rhythm by pausing at the end of the inhalation so as to hold the breath in for a few seconds. The breath should be contained at the level of the diaphragm and the rib-cage, not at the throat. It is more a question of stopping the breath than of holding it in. There should be absolutely no sense of strain or feeling of bursting. Start by holding the breath in for only one second, then build up to three or four very gradually. When you let the breath go again it should be a smooth transition, simply continuing the regular flow. If you find that you are letting the breath out in a gasp, it means that you are holding it for too long or in the wrong way.

Practise deep breathing with inhalation retention for a few cycles, then do a few more cycles of normal deep breathing before relaxing the breath completely.

2   This is a progression of the last exercise. You can try it once you are able to practise the above with ease. The principle is the same, but instead of keeping the breath in at the end of the inhalation only, you pause several times during the inhalation, retaining the breath at each stage. Start the exercise with a long, deep exhalation. Then start the inhalation, pause, hold; continue inhaling, pause, hold; continue, etc., up to four times, ending with a retention; then smoothly exhale again. Listen to the sound of the breath very carefully to make sure that it is even and smooth. Although interrupted, it should not feel or sound jerky.

After completing a few cycles, return to normal deep breathing for a few more cycles, then relax the breath altogether.

Try to practise a few minutes of deep breathing every day, especially towards the end of pregnancy when it is a joy to do, and when the baby really benefits from the boost in oxygen. You can do it at any time, first thing in the morning, or after Savasana when you have been practising the other asanas. When you have finished your breathing practice, lie down on the floor in Savasana for a few minutes, letting the breath and the whole body relax.

*Chapter 7*

# Changes during Pregnancy

'I never suffered from any of the common ailments of pregnancy, I had no backache for example. I'm sure this may well be because of my yoga practice. When practising yoga I always felt very much in touch with my body and with the growing child. Particularly after a class, all my tensions and anxieties would fade away so that I felt totally relaxed and positive about life.'

*Ros*

'I had a very stressful job when I was pregnant, all sorts of people were putting pressure on me. By the regular practice of yoga I found I could contain myself and remain calm throughout a crisis. In fact my boss used to pass any tantrums on to me! I think calmness is the essence of what yoga did for me when pregnant and in this way I felt I was protecting my baby as it grew – I knew that if I was going to go on working, I had to remain calm.'

*Justyne*

'I found the breathing especially useful in this my third pregnancy for I was having so much trouble sleeping. After a yoga session I would sleep more deeply and not suddenly startle awake at two and be unable to sleep for the next three hours.'

*Tessa*

'What I found so inspiring about [the exercises] was that they were so thoroughly grounded in the body. The book explained very clearly the physiology of labour, and how the "exercises" helped to prepare for it – increasing flexibility of the joints, etc. So as I did them I felt I was sensibly preparing myself physically, as far as possible, for the daunting, challenging and exciting task that lay ahead. The more I did them, the more I came to see how much the benefits I got from doing them were mental and psychological as well as physical. . . . I felt in touch with something very ancient and deeply female, a source of strength to help me face the coming labour. For of course labour and birth are not merely athletic feats; they have all sorts of layers of meaning and images attached to them, and I think the psychological preparation for labour is as important as the physical, if not more so. If doing yoga did no more than teach the habit of effective relaxation, it would be worth doing for that reason alone! But when I was doing the "Shakti" Pose, and others, all sorts of images would come into my mind, which were very important, I think now, in preparing me for labour. Images of labour as a leap into the dark, a plunge into the deep end; or at other times, as a narrow passage very similar to the narrow gateway of death that my father had so recently passed through; as a state of transition, a journey into the unknown; an adventure in femaleness.'

*Penny*

# The first three to four months

The first three months of pregnancy are crucial for the healthy formation and development of the baby. The third month sees the end of the embryonic stage, during which everything that will be found in the grown human being is established. By then all the organs, limbs and muscles are formed in miniature and need only to grow and become more refined. It is during the first three months that miscarriage is most likely to occur if it is due to a fault in the foetus' formation.

This early stage is the most 'creative' part of the pregnancy, and the successful formation of the foetus depends to a large extent on the state of health of both parents. Ideally, both should be fit and healthy before conception. During the first three months of pregnancy, it is especially important for the mother to eat well and to take adequate rest. This is usually ensured if a woman listens to her own body – and one of the great benefits of yoga is that it helps to bring us in tune with our bodies, which is important in a culture in which our conditioning tends to alienate us from our physical life. For example, in early pregnancy, most women experience an overwhelming fatigue which is not like any other kind of tiredness. It seems to have little to do with one's everyday output of energy – it is nothing like the tiredness that may come at the end of pregnancy as a result of carrying around considerable extra weight – but seems to be organic, a tiredness that comes from within and has to be endured during this formative and almost parasitic period of the pregnancy. At this stage there is an instinct to surrender to this fatigue and to sleep as much as possible until it passes, usually at around twelve or thirteen weeks, though for some women it disappears sooner, and a few women do not experience it at all.

The same is true of the feelings of nausea which often accompany this stage of pregnancy. Unlike most of the other 'problems' of pregnancy, which can be lessened or avoided altogether by keeping fit, this early nausea does not seem to be a sign that anything is wrong; in fact it has often been interpreted as a sign that the pregnancy is healthy and well established. It does help you to get through this difficult stage if you are instinctively aware that these feelings are 'right' and not a sign of disorder; this is rather like distinguishing in yoga between pain associated with healthy stretching and that associated with injury.

Many women find that they are brought dramatically in touch with their body's needs through the change in their appetite. It is common to suddenly be unable to tolerate alcohol, nicotine, coffee and other substances, some of which are known to be harmful during pregnancy, even if they are normally taken at other times. Smells can provoke as strong a reaction as tastes. Your appetite may increase enormously, or you may develop cravings for particular types of food. As long as you are following a generally healthy diet, it is wise to follow your own appetite and let your body have what it seems to require. It is important to continue to listen attentively to your body's needs and not to dull your awareness by simply getting into the habit of overeating; eat only when you are hungry. You may find that your needs change several times during the course of your pregnancy, so that at one period you may be eating twice as much as you normally do, and at another you may be satisfied with very little.

### Yoga practice in the first few months

Due to tiredness or nausea, you may not feel like practising yoga at this stage. However, it is well worth making the effort to do it; you may discover that it is only while you are practising the asanas that you forget about these feelings. The fact that you are concentrating on the postures helps to take your mind off your condition, but also the act of stretching the body helps to make you feel more alive and to relieve the symptoms. You may find that there are certain postures that are particularly helpful in this respect. In general, all the asanas can be done during the first sixteen weeks – your only limitation may be fatigue. In this case, try to practise mostly in the daytime rather than in the evening, though the calming postures, such as Shoulderstand and forward-bends, can be done just before going to bed. Do practise the standing postures, but if necessary do not hold them for as long as usual. At all stages of pregnancy it is best to start your practice without any preconceptions, for you may be surprised at what you can do once you have begun. Just make sure that you do not push yourself at this time.

Since the foetus is still tiny in the first few months and the uterus, although enlarged, has not yet risen out of the protection of the pelvis, there is no problem about doing the usual range of forward-bends, twists and back-bends which compress, massage and stretch the abdomen. In fact, the improvement in circulation to this area is beneficial. The inverted postures can be done as usual and are particularly valuable at this stage of pregnancy. They help to regulate hormone production, they restore energy and revitalise you, and they help to banish lethargy or depression by giving you literally a new perspective on life. And regular practice of Savasana will be very valuable to you in helping to lessen fatigue and in giving you equanimity.

Since as yet there is no strain on the abdominal and pelvic-floor muscles, this is a good time to exercise them specifically to strengthen them. If your muscles are weak, perhaps as a result of a previous birth, practise the stomach muscle exercises, described in Chapter 9, every day as well as doing your usual yoga practice. Continue these exercises through the first four months or as long as feels comfortable. As strong abdominal work increases internal pressure, this can put a strain on the pelvic-floor muscles if they are not strong. So always, before tightening the abdominal muscles, tighten the pelvic floor. Practising the full range of twisting postures, back-bends and forward-bends helps to keep the stomach muscles in good tone.

One of the first signs of pregnancy is an increase in the size of the breasts, which can be enough to make you more round-shouldered than usual, so practise regularly the shoulder exercises described on pp. 27–34. Svanasana, the Dog Pose, is a wonderful posture to practise from early in pregnancy, to work the shoulders, open the chest, promote deep breathing, stretch the spine and legs, and work the feet. It is a valuable pose to be able to do in later pregnancy, but this will be possible only if you have practised it frequently before you reach that stage.

If you wish to work out a programme for practice during the first four months, make sure that you include the following: the inverted postures, all the standing poses, Svanasana (Dog Pose), one or two back-bends and twisting poses, Paschimottanasana (forward-bend), squatting, and Savasana (Corpse Pose). On the days when you have very little time for practice, then do Svanasana, Headstand (if practised), Sarvangasana (Shoulderstand) and Savasana. And remember to practise your pelvic-floor exercises.

## General exercise in the first few months

If you normally take regular exercise apart from yoga, then continue to do so when you are pregnant. Unless it is an especially strenuous activity, try not to give it up completely because of nausea or tiredness. If you do, you will probably find it difficult to start again later on. Like your practice of the asanas, you may find that the exercise helps to relieve any unpleasant early symptoms, helps you to sleep well and regulates your appetite.

Swimming is especially recommended, since it can be continued right up to the day of birth if wished, it can be done at whatever pace you like, and it is very relaxing as well as invigorating. A good swim always makes you feel lighter and more streamlined. Late in pregnancy, it is a marvellous feeling to have the weight of the baby removed from you by the support of the water; but it is a good idea to start swimming early, or you may feel rather conspicuous if you wait until you are six months pregnant before going to your local baths. Breast-stroke is good for opening the chest and shoulders and stimulating circulation to the pelvic area, and back-stroke is relaxing for the neck.

Fresh air seems particularly important at the early stage of pregnancy, especially if you have any sensations of nausea, for you become as sensitive to smells as to tastes. Walking and cycling (if possible not in the midst of traffic fumes) are very enjoyable and, like swimming, the pace can be varied according to how you feel.

# The middle period, from four to about seven months

This is the time of pregnancy that many women enjoy the most. The advantages of pregnancy are very apparent; for example, you can feel the baby's movements, you probably have plenty of energy, and your skin and hair are in fine, healthy condition. Early fatigue and nausea will have passed, and you are probably not yet big enough to suffer from heartburn or insomnia or to feel burdened with weight. During this time, as the baby grows and becomes more responsive, you become increasingly aware of its movements and reactions to outside stimuli. Certain asanas, especially those which put a good stretch on the abdomen, may cause the baby to kick or move vigorously, as though they are very stimulating to it. The stretching you do in the postures is now directly beneficial to the baby itself, creating more space for movement and supplying more oxygen through the placenta from improved circulation and breathing.

This stage of pregnancy is a good time to start practising deep breathing exercises, if you are not already doing them, and to do plenty of postures which really make space in the front of the body, such as those in which the arms are stretched up above the head. Forward-bends will become more difficult, but can probably still be done with the legs spread apart and with the help of a belt. Certain twists will now have to be discontinued. The standing poses are very enjoyable at this stage, as you probably have plenty of energy and the advantage of supple joints and ligaments, loosened by the pregnancy hormones. The inverted postures can be done as usual, though Sarvangasana (Shoulderstand) becomes more difficult, and Halasana (Plough Pose) must now be done with your feet raised on a chair. As long as you feel happy in Shoulderstand, continue to do it without support, but it is important that you are able to obtain enough lift to keep the front of the body open and unconstricted. As soon as you feel that the baby is squashed, or that breathing is difficult, then start practising with the support of a chair, as described and illustrated on p. 73. Headstand should pose no problems, but from now on it is wise to practise it near a wall, just in case you lose your balance. If you normally move into Headstand with your legs straight, now is the time to start going up with bent knees instead, to avoid straining the abdominal and lower back muscles. You should be getting quite adept at squatting by now, with nicely lengthened muscles in the back of the calves, and supple ankles, and you should be spending a lot of time sitting on the floor. From now on, make sure that you practise at least two of the essential sitting poses every day.

If you have been practising the asanas from the beginning of pregnancy, and especially if you have been doing them since well before conception, you should have none of the problems which often appear at this stage, such as constipation, varicose veins, backache or cramp. However, if any of these do occur, see the tips for dealing with these complaints at the end of this chapter. Be especially aware of your posture at this stage as the abdomen enlarges, and remind yourself of Tadasana every time you find yourself standing still.

For your programme of daily practice, include some standing poses every day;

the inverted postures; Svanasana (Dog Pose); as many sitting postures as possible, including squatting; Savasana (Corpse Pose); deep breathing; pelvic-floor exercises. On days when you have very little time, do Trikonasana, Sirsasana, Sarvangasana, Halasana, Svanasana, Savasana. In addition, sit on the floor in Baddha Konasana and Upavistha Konasana while doing other things, and at odd moments practise your shoulder exercises.

## General exercise in the middle period

You will probably feel like continuing with your usual exercise during this period, and there is every reason to do so. Even if until now you have not been taking any exercise other than yoga, do try at least to walk every day at a pace that is fast enough to make you breathe more heavily than usual. This aerobic exercise will keep you strong and fit, so that when you have to exert yourself, for example walking up long flights of stairs or carrying heavy shopping, you will not feel faint or breathless. You may feel extremely energetic at this stage of pregnancy. However, do not neglect your relaxation every day, in Savasana. Even five minutes is of great benefit, and can often take the place of the much advised afternoon rest.

# Late pregnancy

If you are fit and healthy, you will probably enjoy your pregnancy to the very end, although in the last weeks the rapidly increasing size of the baby can cause some minor problems. The pressure of the uterus on the stomach, diaphragm, rib-cage, bladder and pelvic floor may give you some discomfort, especially at night when trying to make yourself comfortable in bed. The extra weight you are carrying inevitably slows you down somewhat and makes you tired. However, this is a straightforward fatigue which is banished by rest and alleviated by exercise. Also, the changes which take place are so gradual that you tend to adapt to them accordingly. The compensations of feeling your baby move and respond inside you, together with the sense of well-being and serenity that pregnancy usually brings, means that you may not really notice the limitations of your condition until after the baby is born. Then, suddenly, you become light and agile again, with a relief of pressure on the internal organs, and no problems of insomnia.

As long as your legs and back are strong, as long as you are able to make space in your body through stretching, and you are able to relax unnecessary tension, you should be able to carry your baby to the end with a minimum of discomfort. Previous work in the standing postures, plus any aerobic exercise, should be paying off now. You will still benefit from doing the standing poses, though you may find it too strenuous to hold them for as long as you usually do. When practising these poses now, you should concentrate mostly on creating space, on doing them in a 'soft' way, so that not too much physical effort is involved; your body should feel more and more open without losing its steadiness. Done in this way, the standing postures can be a joy to do until the last days of pregnancy. The same is true of Svanasana (Dog Pose) and Sirsasana (Headstand). These are strong poses, but should be done with a sense of quietness and openness. If they become a strain to hold, then discontinue them. Instead of Dog Pose, do the basic stretch shown on p. 14. Stop bending forward if it becomes uncomfortable, if you feel squashed or find it difficult to breathe. Continue with Sarvangasana (Shoulderstand) only while you feel that you are obtaining a good stretch. Even if you have to give up the rest of the inverted poses now, you can still practise Halasana with your legs completely supported (see p. 72). This way of doing it ensures a good position of the spine and plenty of space for the baby, and is very restful and refreshing.

At the very end of pregnancy, you should pay special attention to all the sitting postures, and in particular to the basic ones such as Baddha Konasana, Upavistha Konasana and squatting, which stimulate the pelvic area; the twisting poses; and those postures in which the arms are stretched above the head, creating maximum space in the trunk for relief of pressure and improvement of breathing. In the last weeks of pregnancy, it is very valuable to practise regular deep breathing, both as a preparation for birth and because the last three months sees a very rapid growth in the baby's brain development and the more oxygen it receives the better. Because of this speed of development, it may be very beneficial for the baby if you can take time off to just sit and be in touch with him or her every day.

On days when you have little time for yoga, at least spend a few minutes sitting and breathing, do one or two postures which improve circulation in the legs (either standing, inverted, Svanasana or Virasana), lie down in Savasana, and continue doing pelvic-floor exercises, with the emphasis on relaxation.

*General exercise in late pregnancy*

There is no reason why you should stop taking your usual exercise unless you find it uncomfortable or feel that it is overtiring you. If the baby's head is engaged and pressing down low in the pelvis, it may be uncomfortable to walk, dance or cycle. At this stage the best exercise is swimming, because the weight is taken off you completely and none of your movements can be jerky or jarring. It could be a daily swim which helps you to cope with your increasing bulk, especially during a hot summer, or if your baby is overdue. And if your baby is late in arriving, exercise helps to sustain a positive mental attitude, so that you do not feel that you are 'just' waiting, but carrying on with life as usual.

# Problems of pregnancy

The following problems are often experienced during pregnancy by women who

92

are not very fit. Regular practice of the asanas can prevent them altogether, and can help to alleviate them if they do occur.

### Problems associated with poor circulation

Varicose veins (including piles), swelling of the hands and feet, cramp, aching legs are all a consequence of poor circulation. The inverted poses help all these conditions. For cramp in the legs, also practise Svanasana (Dog Pose) and squatting, which stretch the calf muscles. Virasana (Hero Pose) and Supta Virasana help to relieve varicose veins. In general, sit on the floor in a yogic position rather than on chairs with knees crossed. Take plenty of moving exercise such as walking or swimming.

### Backache

This is usually due to poor posture, weak muscles and pregnancy hormones which soften the ligaments supporting the spine. If you practise yoga regularly, you may never get it, but if you do, lie down on the floor so that the painful area can relax completely. For the lower back, do the pelvic tilting exercise described on p. 107 and Setu Bandha Sarvangasana (Bridging Pose, p. 74). Squatting can give immediate relief. In general, keep your abdominal muscles strong, and pay attention to your posture. For the upper back, do the spine stretch on p. 15 and the shoulder exercises on pp. 27 and 34.

### Problems associated with inactivity and poor breathing

The main complaints here are breathlessness, pain in the ribs, and constipation. If you have trouble with the first two, *stretch* as much as possible. Try the standing poses and those sitting positions in which your arms are stretched above your head. Supta Virasana, with cushions (see p. 60), opens the chest and rib-cage and makes breathing easier. When you practise Savasana, instead of lying flat on the floor, use cushions under your back as in Supta Virasana. Practise deep breathing in a comfortable sitting posture every day.

If you suffer from constipation, practise the inverted poses, the standing poses and, in the earlier months, forward-bends. Keep your abdominal muscles strong and practise deep breathing – sluggish intestines need exercise and massage from stomach muscles and diaphragm. Also, check your diet and make sure that you are taking plenty of fibre and water.

### Heartburn

This is difficult to avoid altogether because the enlarging uterus inevitably presses on the stomach. Stretching is the only answer (see postures recommended for breathlessness, above). Eat little and often, and not too near bed time.

*Insomnia*

This may be due to problems already listed here, but if there is no obvious physical cause, try Sarvangasana (Shoulderstand), supported Halasana (Plough Pose), forward-bends and Savasana (Corpse Pose).

*Chapter 8*

# Labour and Birth

'My son's birth was not easy, but complicated and fairly long, nevertheless a beautiful experience.'

*Kathy*

'Labour can sometimes be arduous and difficult, as was my first labour which lasted 1½ days. Yoga strengthens the body and I wonder if I could have coped as I did if I had been less fit. Yoga affects the whole person, not just the body. It helped me particularly during the births of my second and third children to be "centred" throughout labour and to work in harmony with my body.'

*Ros*

'I was certainly supple enough to kneel right down in the sort of "active birth" position, but I found I resisted doing this during the birth because it speeded up the contractions which were hurting. The birth was so quick in any case that I find it difficult to say whether this was due to yoga. I certainly didn't remain "in control", and I've rather come round to thinking that I don't want to, that I want to shout and writhe around and let my feelings out.'

*Tessa*

'I would say that yoga has a lot to offer pregnant women. Childbirth is a time when the union of "body" and "spirit", head and womb, is not an abstract question, a frivolous metaphysical concern, but a dire practical necessity. If we are not at one with ourselves, labour will be prolonged and unnecessarily stressful.'

*Penny*

'One major contribution yoga made to me was that one learns to work from the inside outwards, which is essential in labour. To be able to "sink into your body", and be aware of what it is experiencing without fear. For example, I was being examined at what turned out to be the onset of the second stage, and found that being on my back was unbearable. I brushed the midwife aside and lunged upright and found immediate relief, as a semi-squatting position made it so much easier for me to handle the overwhelming desire to bear

down. Later I realised that the large size of my baby (11 lbs 10
oz) would have made it almost impossible to push her out from
a supine position. Even in a squat, with the help of gravity,
there was a moment when she appeared to be "stuck".'

*Tonie*

In a sense, it is misleading to separate the phases of childbirth into compartments,
such as early, middle and late pregnancy, first stage of labour, transition and
second stage. Such labels can be useful and necessary, but they should not affect
your expectations and hence your experience of the real thing. When this period of
a woman's life is lived through without preconceptions, it is experienced as a
continuous process, without clearly marked beginnings and endings. Surrendering
to this process and not trying to be always in control of events makes for a more
relaxed pregnancy, birth and post-natal period. Having expectations of how
things should happen only leads to anxiety when they don't. Anticipating birth as
the culmination of pregnancy and the peak on the horizon can lead to a feeling of
anti-climax and depression afterwards. Staying in the present with the help of
yoga, and enjoying every stage for itself as it happens, can give you a wonderful
sense of being a part of the flow and harmony of life.

On the practical level, it is impossible to say where pregnancy ends and labour
begins, at what stage the child in the womb becomes a person, which moment is the
actual point of birth, and so on. The more sensitive you are to your own body, the
more you will probably experience how gradual are the transitions from one stage
to another. There *are* women who find that they suddenly go into labour – after all,
there are cases of women who are unaware that they are pregnant until they find
themselves giving birth – but usually it is felt as a gradual, not a clear-cut,
transition. It is significant that medical books telling how to recognise the onset of
labour cite several different signs, of which not all may be present. The
contractions of the uterus, which are a preparation for the birth, can be felt by
some mothers (especially with second or third pregnancies) as early as the fourth
month, and in fact they do take place from the very beginning. The softening and
even dilating of the cervix can start days or weeks before the birth. The membranes
may break before labour is considered to have really begun, or near the end when
labour is well established, just before the birth of the baby's head. Within a general
pattern there is room for much individual variation, not only from one woman to
another, but also for the same woman from one birth to another. There are always
many factors which influence every event, most of them unknown; the best that
you can do for yourself and your baby is to optimise those that you have some
control over: your own health and state of mind, your helpers, your environment,
and to trust in the unknown.

'Birth can be seen now, not as a procedure separate from the living of each day,
but rather as a *proceeding* from the very roots of it. The greatest preparation
that can be made for the birth of a child is to allow for the constant arising of

birth in one's self. And this arising can take place only in a space that is clear and free of expectation.'

*Maria Rosenstone*

In our society, we seem to have a preoccupation with measuring, labelling and classifying, even when we are dealing with such an unmeasurable experience as birth. The salient facts about any birth – often the first questions asked, and always the facts recorded – are the length of labour, the length of 'first stage' and 'second stage', the speed with which the third stage was completed, the weight and length of the baby, and then the timing of feeds and the intervals between them. In his book, *Genèse de l'Homme Ecologique*, Michel Odent has this to say about demand feeding:

'To encourage a breast feed just after delivery, the first step towards demand feeding, is a typical counter-cultural act. Feeding on demand is perfectly irrational in a commercial society geared to productivity, a society in which all social exchanges are converted into business transactions, a society where time is a commodity, and where one must learn early on how to measure it, that is fragment it.'

Significantly, there are no clocks in his maternity unit.

Thus, to participate fully in birth, whatever kind of birth it turns out to be, to meet the experience and live it through rather than attempting to protect yourself from it by means of drugs or other devices intended to remove you from the experience (even set breathing patterns fulfil this function), it is necessary to let go of certain attitudes and expectations, in fact to let go of any ideas concerning the experience altogether. This should come more easily to those who are accustomed to yoga practice. When there has been a complete opening to an experience, an acceptance of it with nothing in yourself that says 'no', then, however difficult or painful the experience turns out to be, there can be no regrets afterwards, but often a sense of the rightness of the way things happened. The following remarks could apply equally well to your yoga practice and to the way you approach your birth experience. You may find them helpful in colouring your attitude, especially if your surroundings are less than relaxing.

Do not try to *do* anything, only to undo what is stopping you from accepting what is happening in your body.
Take your attention away from your head to the centre of your body to feel grounded and stable.
Release tension on the exhalation.
When a sensation is painful, go towards it, meet it, listen to it. Do not try to interpret it before listening.
Do not impose a posture on your body. Let your body find the posture for itself.

97

Be attentive to the moment, not to a future goal.
Do not force, but cooperate. Do not overpower the body, but let it flow.
Do not act with great force and willpower, but with great clarity and affection.

*Dona Holleman*

Tension constricts the body from the periphery to the centre as when you frown or feel cold. Relaxation opens the body from the centre to the periphery as when you smile, stretch or yawn.

*Dona Holleman*

See if you can become really sensitive to [the contraction] and see what it's trying to tell you to do, see what shape it wants you to take.

*Ina May Gaskin*

Perhaps most important of all:

Your body knows how to do this. Have trust in your body and the way it works.

## Breathing during labour

As when practising the asanas, use the breath to release tension. Do not impose a breathing pattern on the body, but simply stay very aware of the breath, particularly the exhalation. On the exhalation, consciously relax and go with the sensations. Breathe as deeply as you like, but let the breathing follow the body, do not let it reflect a frightened mind. At difficult stages, making noises is very helpful and should not be discouraged. Releasing sound helps to release tension and pain, so do not feel inhibited about moaning, grunting or crying out. However, let it be a natural expression of what is happening in the body, not a cry of frightened anticipation. Try making your noises 'yes' noises rather than 'no' noises.

## Postures for labour

The positions adopted for labour by women who give birth instinctively are mostly upright ones, whether standing, sitting, squatting or kneeling. These postures are physiologically appropriate, since they enlist the help of gravity, they keep the front of the body free, the weight of the uterus off the spine and the major blood vessels which pass through the abdomen, they allow the pelvis to widen without hindrance, they allow the mother to make helpful rocking and swaying movements, and enable her to breathe easily; in fact, they literally keep things moving. If rest is needed, the side lying position is nearly always preferred to lying on the back. Lying on the back, in many places still a feature of hospital birth, is an unnatural and uncomfortable position for labour for several reasons. It tends to slow labour down, contractions being more painful and less efficient; circulation is poor since the uterus presses on the major blood vessels, reducing the supply of oxygen to the baby and possibly causing foetal distress; the pelvis cannot open properly because the sacrum and coccyx are trapped with the weight of the body on them – this can also cause back pain; breathing is difficult and the mother tends to feel submerged and overwhelmed by the experience instead of being alert, 'riding' it; she cannot move her pelvis or trunk easily; and when it comes to pushing, she is working against gravity and lacks the help of the diaphragm and abdominal muscles pressing down on the uterus. Lying on the back is a position of complete stillness, as in Savasana, when one is able to forget about bodily sensations and be aware only of the breath and the state of the mind. Savasana means 'Corpse Pose'. Its very name suggests that it is not a position for bringing life into the world!

When a woman is giving birth, there is no way she can cut herself off from her body; on the contrary, she has to be extremely receptive to all sensations and be totally in her body. And these sensations mostly demand that she move and change position constantly, never staying symmetrical for long, always shifting, rocking, changing her breathing, releasing sound, sometimes clinging to another person for comfort and support. In other words, labour is a time of great restlessness, though not the restlessness of an agitated mind, which is usually reflected in peripheral activity, but a constant movement arising from the centre, a kind of 'dance of creation'. There may be times when a woman in labour is very still and relaxed, usually between contractions, but this is part of the larger pattern of change.

The more easily you are able to move and change position, the more you will be able to meet your body's demands in labour; so this is where your yoga practice stands you in good stead. Your joints will be supple enough to take up whichever position feels most appropriate, and you will have the energy and strength to keep moving for some hours. In early labour it is a good idea to move about as much as possible, in fact to continue your normal activities for as long as you can, whether you are working or playing or out at the shops. There is no magic point at which you are suddenly in labour and have to down tools. Think of yourself as an active person who just happens to be in labour. This way the contractions will be less noticeable and more efficient. As the contractions start to get stronger, so that you really need to concentrate on them, stop whatever you are doing just while they last and rest against something or someone, leaning forward – you will probably do this naturally anyway. The uterus tilts forward as it contracts, so if you lean forward there is no resistance from gravity. Other positions which are usually comfortable in early labour are sitting cross-legged or in Baddha Konasana, with your weight on your buttock bones and your spine lifting; squatting on a low stool, or on the floor leaning on to your hands; and kneeling, either upright or leaning forward against something. If you are on a hospital bed, you can sit cross-legged on it, or sit on the edge with your feet resting on a high stool by the bed.

As you go into stronger labour and find yourself needing to concentrate and turn inwards more and more, you may find yourself using the kneeling position during contractions. A very helpful kneeling posture is that with the knees spread apart, leaning forward against a bed, a chair or a pile of cushions. It has been pointed out that the kneeling posture is a position of prayer, in which the mind can be in a highly concentrated, meditative state. This state of consciousness becomes more and more necessary as the sensations of birth gain momentum – they cannot easily be borne with your everyday mind, and it can seem a violence at this stage for your attendants to speak to you in ways that require you to answer using your rational brain; only touch, physical support and comforting noises are appropriate. However, between contractions, you may be amazed to find that you are sitting up again, feeling as though nothing unusual is going on and chatting to those around you! As the birth approaches, these intervals of relaxation become shorter and shorter. At this stage it is important not to be persuaded to lie down on your back, for example, if the midwife wants to do an internal examination, for once there it is extremely difficult to get up again, and you may be overwhelmed and lose touch with your body altogether. At the end of the first part of labour, just before the pushing contractions begin, it is very hard for most of us to surrender to the sensations entirely and feel at one with the process, especially if there is any outside disturbance. It can be helpful here to bear in mind that your body is telling you that you are nearly there, you really do not have far to go before you are pushing your baby out. It is easy for fear to enter at this point – 'I can't cope with this much longer, what if it gets worse?' – but when you have reached this point, there will not *be* much longer. All too often in hospitals drugs have been given near the end of labour quite unnecessarily, too late to be of any use, because of panic on the part of the mother and the attendants; and the drugs go straight to the baby.

Once the pushing contractions begin, and there is no mistaking when the pushing urge overtakes you, then it is most helpful to be in an upright position (unless the delivery is very fast, when the all-fours posture may be preferred). Squatting has the great advantage that it opens the pelvis to its widest and is the easiest position in which to release the pelvic-floor muscles. For most people, it is more comfortable to be supported in the squatting position, so that the thighs can be relaxed, either by one person holding from behind, or by two people, one on each side. For more information on birth positions, see the books mentioned in the reading list.

When the placenta is ready to be delivered, it will simply fall out on its own if you stay in the squatting or semi-squatting position. In the meantime, you will probably find your yoga sitting positions useful for holding and feeding your baby, unless you are very tired or the perineum is very sore.

## Interventions in the birth

The value of yoga lies in helping us not to disturb the natural working of the body through fear or tension; it helps us to undo the blocks that may stand in the way of a natural, normal, safe birth. All intervention disturbs this process. By intervention is meant any obtrusive procedure which attempts to transfer control of the birth from the mother's own body and instincts to those 'managing' the delivery. Into this category fall the following: induction or acceleration of labour, insistence on the mother lying in bed, intrusive examinations, withholding food and drink, foetal monitoring by machines which have to be attached to mother or baby, pain-killing drugs, forceps, episiotomy, injection of drugs to speed delivery of placenta, immediate cutting of umbilical cord, separation of baby from mother after birth. (The list is not exhaustive.) Of course, some of these procedures are occasionally necessary for medical reasons and can be life-saving; but the instances where they are really necessary, where the natural process, if allowed to unfold, would result in catastrophe, are rare. The sad thing is that all forms of intervention listed above have become a matter of routine for most hospital births, they are applied indiscriminately, demeaning not only the whole experience of birth, but also the true value of technology. The woman who wants a natural birth, especially if she is a first-time mother, has to be extremely wary of any procedure that is carried out on her, even if it seems a simple matter of routine, unless she has complete trust in those attending her and knows that they are aware of and in sympathy with her wishes. For it can take only one intervention to disturb the natural process to the extent that further intervention is needed. A typical example is the induction of labour on the grounds that the baby is statistically overdue. Induced births are nearly always much quicker and more painful than normal ones and it is usual for the mother to request pain relief by pethidine or epidural. These drugs can interfere with her responses so that the pushing urge does not establish itself properly and episiotomy and forceps may be deemed necessary. Drugs taken by the mother may also adversely affect the baby's breathing after the birth, necessitating resuscitation and sometimes injection of an antidote into the newborn baby. The induced baby may even turn out to be premature. This means separation of mother and baby immediately after the birth, and then possibly problems for the mother with breast feeding because of the traumatic experience, and pain from stitches in the perineum. It is this 'snow-ball effect' that makes the apparently well-meaning administrations of 'something for the pain', or 'just a little cut to help the baby out' so insidious. And many women are not even informed about the procedures that are carried out on their bodies, let alone asked for their permission. Remember, you cannot improve on a natural birth.

There are some excellent publications available which will inform you on the nature and implications of medical procedures at birth, and these are listed on p. 113. In general, try to build up a good relationship with your midwives and doctor during pregnancy and discuss your ideas with them; keep yourself fit and healthy through your yoga practice and a good diet; have a person you love and trust with you during labour both for support and as an intermediary between you and the professionals if needed; try to make sure that your environment is as calm and relaxing as possible – no strangers coming and going during labour; and be prepared to do your own thing: this is your birth, your baby, one of the most important times of your life, you have every right to do it your way. It is not a time to be afraid of 'making a fuss' if necessary, but with the right attitudes and a bit of luck, you may not even have to!

The whole matter of the management of labour is really a question not of techniques and procedures, but of deeply rooted attitudes. There is a growing number of people who are concerned at the way in which the individual has lost touch with his or her sense of personal power, surrendering it to the 'experts', to the institution and to the general dictates of society. An area where this is particularly keenly felt is that of birth, where there can be a vast discrepancy between the desires and experience of the individual and the standard medical attitude. According to the latter, the process of birth is a mainly mechanical operation, fraught with risks which can and should be prevented or remedied by purely physical means. The emphasis is on intervention and control. The emotional experience of birth is seen as a luxury, the icing on the cake, which should not be allowed to take precedence or get in the way of the safe and efficient management of the birth.

However, for many people, it is not possible to separate the physical from the emotional, intuitive and spiritual aspects of the self; it is necessary for all to be in harmony for the safe and good outcome of the birth of their child. They are in touch with an instinctive part of themselves which enables them to trust in the natural process. These people will feel safer giving birth in their own home, away from the threat of disturbance and routine medical intervention. It is not the tools themselves they fear, but the attitudes of those wielding them. To be uncompromisingly in favour of natural birth is to have an attitude that is radically different from the accepted way of looking at things in our society; it is what Michel Odent refers to as a counter-cultural act. For this reason, because it requires a complete shift in view-point, any reforms in this direction seem both overwhelmingly simple and overwhelmingly difficult. However, there is room for optimism since, if you can retain your own vision and integrity, with the confidence that your yoga practice can give you, your own personal power and influence can be strong, even if it is not immediately apparent to yourself. Your own example is more potent than any method of force or persuasion.

The following words are by Maria Rosenstone, mother and yoga practitioner, and are taken from Frédérick Leboyer's book, *Inner Beauty, Inner Light*:

A natural birth is a manifestation of spontaneous expression and cannot be schooled, urged or thrust upon a mode of living that is not natural. It requires only a clear channel, a body in health, a mind in understanding, a whole being that is totally open. When the intelligence of the body is awakened, as through the practice of yoga, it will guide the woman throughout the pregnancy, making her feel perhaps more in touch with herself than ever before. She is then close to her own nature and ready to flow with the movement of birth when it begins.

*Chapter 9*

# After the Birth

'After the birth I recovered very quickly which may partly be due to its brevity, but also I think perhaps to having been active and supple right up to the birth.'

*Tessa*

'From birth my son was very lively and open-eyed. I suppose the main benefit I noticed with yoga was the speed with which I recovered and was able to cope with a newborn. The breast feeding was easy and the milk plentiful. I continued to breast feed my son for 2½ years, without feeling unduly tired, a fact I attribute to a daily yoga practice.'

*Kathy*

'After the births I felt very energetic and healthy and my body soon got back to normal.'

*Ros*

'Immediately after the birth I weighed exactly the same as before I was pregnant, my tummy went back to normal, I had no stretch marks. I think the suppleness that practising yoga gives you is very important.'

*Justyne*

'After the birth yoga made me very aware of my posture, especially when carrying the baby. I used to sit cross-legged when feeding which I really enjoyed and I suffered no backache. I had no problems with breast feeding.'

*Fran*

'Labour began and two hours later I had the baby! I felt my body functioned really well, I pushed the baby out easily, I felt very strong. I really enjoyed my birth at home and felt yoga helped me. I was up and about very easily and healed very quickly compared with my other two births. There were no problems with breast feeding either.'

*Sally*

'Yoga helped in the post-natal period physically and mentally. My body healed quickly from a large tear and I was soon mobile and coping with my enlarged family.'

*Tonie*

'I had a very healthy pregnancy and kept very fit throughout. Unfortunately the birth of my daughter was long and complicated and after a two-week stay in hospital, it was several months before I started to recover. It was during this time that I felt I needed some form of exercise, of movement to try and regain my fitness and particularly to put behind me the trauma that I had experienced.

'I started Iyengar Yoga classes, this seemed a very gentle way of gradually steering my body, and particularly my state of mind, into a positive direction. I was pleasantly surprised at how soon I started to feel the benefit of yoga, postures that at first seemed almost impossible became a challenge, then a reward. It pleased me to know that I was putting vital energy back into me at a time when I needed it most.

'There were of course some weeks when I felt too tired to cope with a two-hour yoga class and just wanted to sleep instead, but I made myself go, knowing that at the end of class finishing with a relaxation period would do me more good than resting at home. I would leave class feeling bright eyed and rejuvenated, glad that I had gone – had accomplished this state of well-being, and leaving me ready to face the day and anything else.

'I made sure that I never missed a class no matter how tired I felt. In fact the more tired I was, the more I seemed to benefit from yoga.'

*Stephanie*

During the weeks and months after your baby is born, you will really appreciate the benefits of having practised yoga throughout pregnancy. The earlier you started making yourself fit, the more quickly and easily your body will return to its non-pregnant state. This does not mean that you should expect to be 'back to normal' in a matter of weeks; after all, you are now entering a different phase of relationship with your child which is as unique as pregnancy and a continuation of it. During the breast-feeding period, the baby continues to be nourished through a very close bond with you, the mother. The first weeks after the birth are rather like the first weeks of pregnancy in that the changes taking place in the body are extremely rapid. This can make you feel turbulent and unbalanced unless you are able to flow with the process as with the pregnancy and birth, and enjoy each stage for itself. If you continue to practise your yoga and look after yourself intelligently, you will be able to ride the changes with equanimity. Yoga is about skilful living and we need to steer a fine course between neglecting ourselves by ignoring our special condition, and making heavy weather of it by becoming excessively pre-occupied with it.

The post-natal advantages of practising yoga are many. In the first place, you are unlikely to have needed an episiotomy at birth, so you will have avoided all the pain and discomfort of stitches and the problems this can cause with breast feeding, with your ability to relax, and with the sexual relationship. Problems associated with episiotomy can last for a year after the birth. A tear, on the other hand, usually heals much more quickly. Even if you have had an episiotomy, you will probably heal more quickly than usual, since yoga improves the body's capacity to heal itself.

With the help of yoga, all the post-natal changes in the body take place normally and efficiently. The uterus returns to its normal size and position quickly (this is also helped by breast feeding), the pelvic-floor and abdominal muscles are not over-stretched and soon regain their tone, the circulation of hormones in the body is well regulated so that there is a good milk supply, healthy functioning of all the internal organs, and emotional stability. The confidence in your own body, which was so valuable to you during the birth, is of equal value while breast feeding becomes established. You are not likely to have any doubts about your ability to produce enough milk for your child, since you know that your body is in good condition and 'knows' how to do it. And in your relationship with your baby, you will be able to rely on your instincts, you will not doubt your ability as a mother and become vulnerable to the mass of conflicting ideas on how to bring up children that reaches you in the form of books, magazines and advice from friends and professionals. For, in the same way that women are no longer expected to be able to give birth naturally without medical help, new mothers are not expected to know how to care for their own babies without professional guidance. The following lines, taken from a popular book on pregnancy and birth, are indicative of this attitude:

> the babies are together with their mothers a lot during the day for feeding and also so that the mothers can learn how to care for them. Nurses carefully show what should be done.... Four to six days after delivery the mother is generally allowed to go home. Now she will have to manage without help from nurses and doctors.

In hospital, this attitude transmits itself to the new mother, so that unless she can stay in touch with her own instincts, her confidence can be seriously undermined. This is less likely to happen after a home birth, since in her own home a woman does not relinquish responsibility to a person in authority. The midwife makes a daily visit to check the mother's and baby's health and to give support and advice, but she does not take charge.

For first-time mothers, the transition to motherhood is sometimes seen as a psychological problem, in that it can be difficult to adapt to the new role of mother. This problem can only arise if you have a fixed image of yourself in a particular role. The practice of yoga tends to alter this way of seeing yourself; you no longer have any need of a role for your sense of identity, so there is no mental construct which has to be painfully changed or let go of.

# Yoga practice after the birth

You may well be reaping the benefits of your previous yoga practice during pregnancy, but it is important to keep up at least a minimum of practice after your baby is born. You will probably find that you are still carrying your baby with you a great deal of the time, and in ways which can put more strain on your body than carrying it inside you, so you have to pay attention to the way you use your body at this stage. Be as aware of your posture as you were during pregnancy. Carrying your baby in your arms or in a sling can pull your shoulders forward in a rounded position, and can make your posture lopsided if you always carry your baby on the same side. Immediately after the birth, ligaments and tissues are still softened and some muscles are very stretched, so it is important to keep your body in good alignment to avoid strain. Make sure that you sit in a balanced, comfortable position while feeding your baby. You spend a lot of time feeding in the first few weeks, and if you sit with your spine and shoulders collapsed and hunched, this can permanently affect your posture and cause stiffness and pain. The best way to sit for feeding is on the floor in a cross-legged position, with a pillow on your knees to lift the baby to the right height, so that you do not have to stoop forwards.

Relaxation is especially important after your baby is born. You will be tired at first, from the upheaval that your body has been through as well as from broken nights feeding your baby. Fatigue can interfere with your ability to relax, so daily practice of Savasana can be of great value in stopping you from feeling tense, irritable or depressed. Your yoga practice has to be adapted to suit your new way of life, and you will probably have to be very selective about which asanas to include due to lack of time to yourself.

In the first few days after the birth you will probably spend a lot of time resting in bed, and this is an ideal opportunity to start exercising the pelvic-floor muscles. Apart from general stretching of the limbs and deep breathing, the pelvic-floor exercises are the most important ones to concentrate on at first. Do them several times a day, as described on p. 75, with the emphasis now very much on drawing up and tightening the muscles. If you have a cut or tear in the perineum, these exercises will help the healing process since they improve circulation to the area. There is no danger of stitches bursting, since you are drawing them in closer rather than pushing them outwards. It is important to strengthen the pelvic floor before starting strong abdominal muscle exercises, since these place extra strain on the pelvic-floor muscles.

The following are some simple, basic post-natal exercises which should be done during the first week after the birth, and can all be done on a firm bed.

## Abdominal wall tightening

Lying down or sitting, place your hands lightly on your abdomen, just to feel what you are doing, and, on a deep exhalation, slowly and strongly pull in your stomach muscles, after first tightening the pelvic floor. Relax, breathing in. Repeat several times. This simple exercise can be continued for weeks and months after the birth, at any time, whenever you happen to think of it, and if done often enough is surprisingly effective.

## Pelvic tilting

Lying on your back with your knees bent up, breathe out as you tilt your pelvis back so as to flatten your lower back on to the bed or floor. On your next exhalation, contract your pelvic-floor and abdominal muscles. Place a hand above the pubic bone to feel the muscles working. Hold for a few seconds with normal breathing, then relax. Repeat several times.

## Bridging

Lying on your back with your knees bent up, tighten your abdominal and buttock muscles as you gently lift your pelvis from the bed or floor. Don't arch your back.

## Relaxing on your front

Lying on your front not only feels delicious after the months of pregnancy, but also helps the uterus and other pelvic organs to return to their normal position. Place a pillow under your hips (two pillows if your bed is soft) to avoid arching the small of the back. If your breasts are tender place more pillows under your head and shoulders. Rest in this position as often as possible.

## Curl-ups (1)

Lying on your back, bend your knees up, keeping your feet flat on the bed or floor, hip width apart. Keep your pelvis tilted back so that your lumbar spine stays flat on the bed. Breathing out, lift up your head, shoulders, and upper back, then slowly lie back again. Work smoothly, and repeat several times.

## Curl-ups (2)

Lying on your back, straighten both legs and flex your feet so that your toes point upwards. Lift your head until you can see your feet. Repeat several times.

## Leg stretching

Lying on your back, with knees bent up and back flat, straighten and bend up each leg alternately. Then straighten and bend both legs together. Keep the lower back flat on the floor or bed all the time.

Continue with these basic exercises for the first few weeks after the birth, gradually phasing them out as you resume your normal yoga practice. The exercises are most effective if you start them within twenty-four hours of the birth, and keeping up the habit of exercise (even if only five or ten minutes a day) is very helpful in leading you back to a regular yoga session. Try not to stop practising yoga altogether, or it will be more difficult to start again later on, and your body will feel very stiff. You can and should practise Savasana (Corpse Pose) and a little deep breathing from the first day after the birth. Then, as soon as you are up and dressed and back to your normal activities, do a few basic asanas every day, even if you do not manage to set aside much time for yoga. One way of doing this is to wear loose, comfortable clothes all the time (such as track-suits), so that whenever you think of it you can stretch your spine and your legs in the basic stretches, or you could do a couple of standing postures. You can also sustain the habit of sitting on the floor for many activities, especially for feeding, changing and playing with your baby. Make a point of doing your shoulder exercises (p. 27 and 34) at odd moments when your arms are free, and relax in Uttanasana several times a day, especially if you feel tension building up in your head, neck, shoulders or back.

## Postures to practise after the birth

*First six weeks*

| | |
|---|---|
| Standing poses: | Basic stretches (pp. 13–17) |
| | Tadasana |
| | Trikonasana |
| | Virabhadrasana II and Parsvakonasana |
| | Svanasana |
| Forward bends: | Uttanasana |
| | Paschimottanasana |
| | Janu Sirsasana |
| | Triang Mukhaikapada Paschimottanasana |
| | Ardha Baddha Padma Paschimottanasana |

The forward bends strengthen the abdomen, uterus and other internal organs after the birth, and feel marvellous now that the baby is no longer in the way.

| | |
|---|---|
| Shoulder exercises: | Gomukasana |
| | Parsvottanasana |
| | Shoulder Exercise in Uttanasana |
| Sitting poses: | Baddha Konasana |
| | Upavistha Konasana |
| | Virasana |

Wait until bleeding has stopped before doing inverted postures. In the meantime, do Upavistha Konasana lying on your back with legs against wall, and Savasana.

## Six weeks to three months

As well as the above, do as many standing postures as you have time for. Do Sarvangasana every day; it feels marvellous after pregnancy. Also do Sirsasana if you want to. Introduce twisting poses and postures which strengthen abdomen and lower back muscles (such as Jathara Parivartanasana, Navasana).

## Paschimottanasana and Janu Sirsasana

Can now be done by completing the forward bending movement, taking the ribs to the thighs and the head to the knees or shins, as illustrated for the next two forward bending poses.

## Triang Mukhaikapada Paschimottanasana

Sit in Dandasana and bend one leg back as for Virasana. Pull out the flesh from the buttocks using your hands and sit firmly and evenly on the two buttock bones. If you roll over to the side of the straight leg, place a folded blanket under the hip on that side to keep you stable. Reach forward to grasp your foot or ankle with both hands, then, exhaling, rotate the pelvis and stretch forward so as to rest your lower ribs on your thigh and your head on your knee or shin. If possible, clasp your hands beyond the outstretched foot. Relax into the position with normal breathing, then inhale as you sit up, bringing your head up first. Repeat with the other leg bent back.

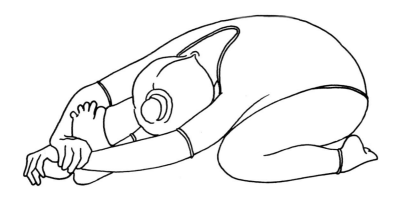

**9.1**  Triang Mukhaikapada Paschimottanasana

*Note*: do not take your head to your knee by bending at the waist and humping your back. Keep the front of your body well stretched and aim to take your lower ribs to your thigh before taking your head down.

109

## *Ardha Baddha Padma Paschimottanasana*

Sit in Dandasana. Place one leg in Padmasana (Lotus) as described on page 56). Keep the other leg outstretched. Reach forward to grasp the foot or ankle of the outstretched leg with both hands, then proceed into the forward bend as described above. Try to stretch so that your lower ribs lift over the foot in Lotus and rest on the thigh, as shown. Repeat on the other side.

Not for beginners.

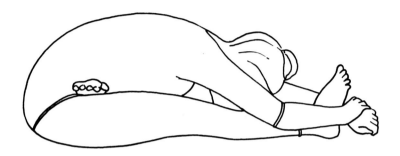

**9.2**  Ardha Baddha Padma Paschimottanasana

## *Shoulder Exercise in Uttanasana*

Stand with your feet parallel, hip width apart, and interlock your fingers behind your back. Exhaling, bend forward from the hips as in Uttanasana, straightening your arms and stretching them up and over your head as far as they will go (palms facing your back, knuckles outwards). Relax your neck. Inhale as you stand up, lifting your head first. Repeat with your fingers interlocked the other way (opposite thumb nearer to you, still with palms facing inwards).

## *Jathara Parivartanasana*

Lie down on your back with legs straight and arms stretched out at shoulder level, palms up. With an exhalation, raise both legs until they are vertical, taking care not to arch your back; flatten your lower back into the floor. Swivel both hips to your left, so that your toes face towards your right. Keep both legs straight throughout. Exhaling, lower your legs to the right so that your feet rest on the floor near to your right hand. Breathe normally and keep your left shoulder flat on the floor. If this is difficult, tether your left arm and shoulder by gripping a piece of heavy furniture with your left hand. Now, exhaling, raise both legs together to the vertical position, keeping them straight. Try not to tense your face, throat or shoulders. Repeat to the other side, then lower your legs to the floor in the starting position and relax completely.

This exercise can be done two or three times in succession.

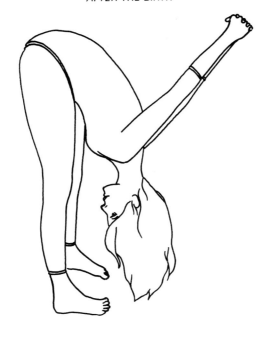

**9.3**  Parvatasana

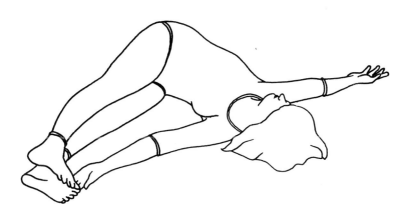

**9.4**  Jathara Parivartanasana

## *Navasana, Boat pose*

Sit in Dandasana, making sure that you are sitting well forward on your buttock bones and lifting your lower back well. Placing your fingertips on the ground beside you for balance, exhale as you raise both legs from the floor, keeping them straight. Do not point your toes. Now stretch your arms out in front of you, palms facing each other. Hold with relaxed breathing, then return to Dandasana. Repeat two or three times.

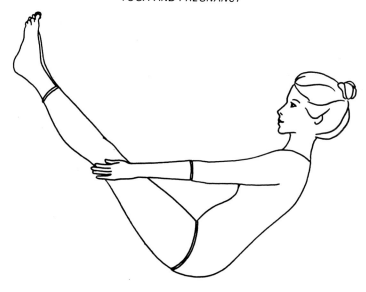

**9.5** Navasana

*Note*: your body should make a V-shape, with straight legs and straight back. Try not to collapse on to the base of your spine, but stretch and lift the lower back. This asana strengthens this area of the back, as well as the stomach muscles. If it is very difficult for you at first, you can practise it with your feet resting on a bed or a chair.

### After three months

Back to normal and your usual yoga practice.

# Reading List

## Yoga Classics

*The Bhagavad Gita*, translated by Juan Mascaro, Penguin Books.
*Aphorisms of Yoga (the Yoga Sutras)*, by Bhagwan Shree Patanjali, translated by Shree Purohit Swami, Faber & Faber.
There is a new translation by Kofi Busia, called *The Gift, The Prayer, The Offering*, Oxford Ashram Publications.
*Light on Yoga*, by B. K. S. Iyengar, Allen & Unwin.

## Birth

*Birth Without Violence*, by Frédérick Leboyer, Fontana/Collins.
*Entering the World – The Demedicalisation of Childbirth*, by Michel Odent, Marion Boyars.
*Childbirth With Insight*, by Elizabeth Noble, Houghton Mifflin Co., Boston, Mass. A fresh approach to preparation for childbirth, acknowledging the unity of body and mind. A superb book, of special value to ante-natal teachers.
*Birthrights – A Parents' Guide to Modern Childbirth*, by Sally Inch, Hutchinson. Packed with information. Outlines in detail all the hospital childbirth procedures, explaining the disadvantages and risks associated with each and arguing against their routine use.
*Birth Issues and Alternatives*, edited by Ros Claxton, Allen & Unwin.
*Birth at Home*, by Sheila Kitzinger, Oxford University Press.
*Spiritual Midwifery*, by Ina May Gaskin, The Book Publishing Co. (USA).

## Preparing for birth

*Inner Beauty, Inner Light*, by Frédérick Leboyer, Collins. Beautiful photographs of Iyengar's daughter practising asanas shortly before the birth of her child.
*Essential Exercises for the Childbearing Year*, by Elizabeth Noble, John Murray. Cannot be too highly recommended. Contains clear physiological explanations of need for exercise during pregnancy. Encourages women to understand their bodies and take responsibility for their own health.
*Exercises for Childbirth*, by Barbara Dale and Johanna Roeber, Century. A simple and inspiring book with lovely photographs. Exercises are based on yoga principles and suitable for anyone. Includes sections on swimming or water exercises, relaxation, massage, a guide to labour, and post-natal exercises.
*Active Birth*, by Janet Balaskas, Unwin Paperbacks. A very useful book which explains the anatomy of pregnancy and birth, with yoga-based exercises for pregnancy and after and much on the birth itself, with birth accounts from many women.

*The Good Birth Guide*, by Sheila Kitzinger, Penguin Books. A guide to hospitals throughout the country based on experiences of women who have given birth in them.

*Good Food Before Birth*, by Cate Lewis, Unwin Paperbacks.

*How to Avoid an Unnecessary Episiotomy*, by Sophy Hoare and Melody Weig.

*The Use of Painkilling Drugs in Labour and What You Need to Know About Them*, by Gerlinde Wilberg.

*Getting the Kind of Birth You Want in Hospital*, by Ros Claxton.

*Home Birth Information Sheet* These and other leaflets published by the Birth Centre London, 101 Tufnell Park Road, London N7. Send a s.a.e. for an information sheet. A *Yoga Poster* showing twenty asanas for pregnancy in clear black and white photographs (size 25″ × 18″) is also available.

# Index